T0198759

Playing

with

Cancer

AT AGE 13

© 2020 Aditi Goel. All rights reserved.

No part of this book may be reproduced, stored in a retrieval system, or transmitted by any means without the written permission of the author.

AuthorHouse™
1663 Liberty Drive
Bloomington, IN 47403
www.authorhouse.com
Phone: 1 (800) 839-8640

Because of the dynamic nature of the Internet, any web addresses or links contained in this book may have changed since publication and may no longer be valid. The views expressed in this work are solely those of the author and do not necessarily reflect the views of the publisher, and the publisher hereby disclaims any responsibility for them.

This book is printed on acid-free paper.

ISBN: 978-1-7283-4062-3 (sc)
ISBN: 978-1-7283-4063-0 (e)

Print information available on the last page.

Published by AuthorHouse 01/22/2020

authorHOUSE

Playing

with

Cancer

AT AGE 13

ADITI GOEL

Contents

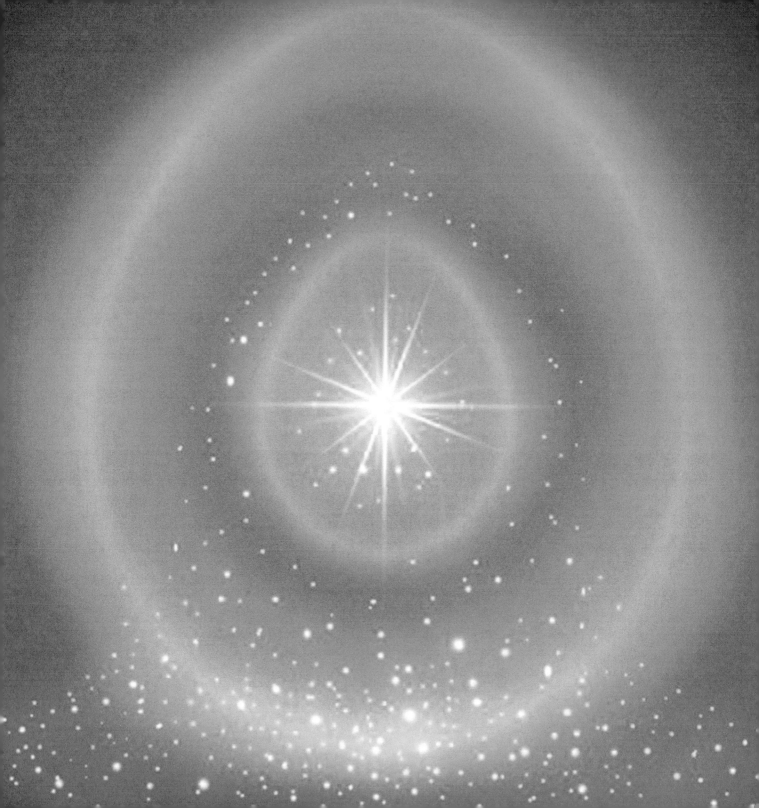

Foreword

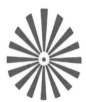

It isn't often that I encounter a profoundly moving story that brings me to tears and elates my spirit. To travel through Aditi's mind and experience how this young, amazing girl viewed her cancer and her treatment at the age of 13 will awaken and empower anyone going through the reality of this disease.

This book, Playing with Cancer, will also enlighten the caregivers and all who face any life-threatening challenge on their journey of life. Imagine traveling through a portal of innocence that offers you a unique perspective? She offers such insight into the separation of the body and soul, and the force that inner silence can have on the healing process. Her victory over cancer is a testament of what the power of the mind can do. She reminds us to keep looking into the future being bright and not get stuck on what's broken.

Playing with Cancer will inspire any reader to remember playing with life as it unfolds is the only way to go! This is a must read and a gift to our world.

Sister Dr. Jenna
BrahmaKumaris Meditation Museum
Host, America Meditating Radio

Introduction

When I was 13 years old, I was diagnosed with cancer after a germ cell tumor was discovered in my ovary. This was not my family's first encounter with a life-threatening disease. My mother survived stomach cancer shortly before I was born. Four years later, in 2003, she received another dire diagnosis, this time cancer of the blood. She died of the disease when I was not yet four years old.

The aim of writing this book is to tell my story, in all of my different phases of life. I will start off with talking about my family. My family is very small and simple: just my father, my two older brothers, and myself since my mother's death in 2004. My father works as an attorney of law, which he practices in the Supreme Court in Delhi and the High Court in Chandigarh. Both of my brothers live in the United States. The oldest works as a computer engineer, and the younger is a lawyer, like our father. We may not live under the same roof or even on the same continent, but we share a bond distance cannot break. Throughout the many stages of my life, in both good times and bad, my father and my brothers have always been there sharing the journey with me.

My father and I lived in the United States for a time as well. He took a two-year sabbatical to work with the School of Law at University of North Carolina, Chapel Hill I joined an elementary school there to study third and fourth grade. I fondly remember my teachers and classmates from those years. Though it was difficult to leave them and return to DPS Chandigarh in fifth grade, the teachers at my school in India also made me feel comfortable when I returned. Learning to adapt to different situations, living in a variety of places, made it easier to cope with the changes after I was diagnosed with cancer.

There is a familiar adage that says, "Our happiness multiplies on spreading, and our sorrow gets divided on doing the same." I believe very much in this statement. Having a network of close friends and family members by my side during my treatment was one of the key reasons I was able to get through it with my spirits high. In writing this book I want to say a heartfelt thank you to every doctor and nurse who was part of my treatment, every family friend who opened their homes and hearts to us, and all the others whose love kept me strong through my ordeal. I am forever grateful to everyone who is mentioned in the story that follows.

This book aims to share my personal views on my experiences with cancer. I feel proud that I've been able to achieve a victory over the deadly disease. The treatment and support I received were instrumental, of course, but just as important was that I had a spirit to live. It was this spirit that made me keep fighting even when things were painful and difficult, and this spirit I want to emphasize in the story that follows. Though I almost reached a dead end, I rebounded and got back up with a bang. My story is not one of struggle but one of strength and hope, from my unusual conception through my surgery, chemotherapy, and recovery.

It was my father who convinced me to write this book as a way to tell my story and express my views. A few years have passed since the end of my treatment and it feels like the right time to share my experiences. The inspiring stories of the Indian cricket player Yuvraj Singh and the Bollywood superstar Manisha Koraila, who had also beaten cancer, motivated me to tell my story.

I hope my narrative shall encourage other people to find their own spirit and inner strength. Cancer affects people all over the world, of all ages, races, and walks of life. Every survivor has their own unique story of how they traveled from diagnosis through treatment to remission. This book tells my personal journey.

My Support Base

Swami Debananda ji: Swamji is a saint of the Vedic order based in Burdwan, West Bengal. Though a deeply spiritual holy man, Swamiji has not created any cult and does not insist his disciples follow any particular way of worship. At the age of two, I was in mother's lap when I received His first blessings. Thereafter, my contact with Swamiji have been almost regular. Whenever I visit him, it is a unique experience that helps in my spiritual development.

My father: I understand it is usual with every parent to be with their children in every situation and that as a matter of responsibility they provide you everything you need without asking. My father is no different. Although a litigator by profession, I always had a preemptory right over his time, and I did not have to ask for it. To be around me is his first priority. I never visualized my life without him. His huge social capital helped him to successfully manage my illness, my mother's illness and her early departure from this world.

My older brothers: Abhishek and Abhinav

Older than me by 17 years, I call Abhishek Sonu bhaiya. From the beginning, Sonu Bhaiya focused on my development as a logical person and does not believe in spoon feeding. If I am in need, he will provide guidance for me to steer my own vehicle. When it comes to helping me, he follows the American adage: "do not give him a fish, make him to learn fishing." He is an epitome of knowledge and keeps sharing with me every aspect of my life.

I address Abhinav, older than me by 13 years, as Abbu Bhaiya. Since my birth, I always felt Abbu Bhaiya standing with me, no matter the physical distance. Sonu Bhaiya was already away to America when I was born, so Abbu Bhaiya helped take care of me until his departure to US in 2005. We share our visits to religious persons and places like Swami Debanand Ji, Rama Krishna Mission Ashram, Brahma Kumaris, and various popular Sikh Temples like Golden Temple, Anandpur Saheb, Washington DC Gurudwara. He keeps suggesting different books. I liked reading *Snacks for the Soul* by J P Vaswani, a collection of stories that offer emotional, intellectual and spiritual nourishment. As a law student, he would discuss with me small cases full of fun giving me ideas of lawyers' work. Recently he got married to Dr. Nishtha Mehta and I was introduced to her family a while back. On our very first encounter, we developed an instant bond and felt as if we had always known each other.

Both of my brothers are towering personalities in my life. Because of our age difference, I am more like a daughter to both of them than a younger sister. They serve me new delicacies and show me different places of attraction in America. Three of us stay in touch with one another on almost daily basis. I keep sharing my medals and achievements, they keep telling me about anything new happening in their life—and we never fight.

Mr. Ram Singla: He is my father's friend from prior to their marriages. My dad relies upon him very heavily and always values his association. He was the key "family hand" during my mother's illness. Whenever there was any administrative or admissions issue concerning DPS—prior to or after my illness—Ram uncle would take care of them.

Mr. B.K. Singla: He is the elder brother of Mr. Ram Singla, and has always treated my father like his brother, as well. He and his wife, Mrs. Shalu Singla, have always been like parents and mentor to my parents. The family hosted for me a surprise 13th birthday dinner after my surgery. He firmly supported the decision for my treatment to be in USA irrespective of the costs. When we went to the US for post-surgery treatment, Bal uncle joined us a week later and stayed with us until a decision was made for me to do my chemo at Hershey.

Dr. Ram Goel: He is as close to the family as the above two mentioned. He always supported my dad in sending my brothers to the US for higher education, and helped convince my mother to agree to it, as well. He sent me to summer camps at Harrisburg Academy and introduced me to the faculty and the principal there. Being a US citizen, he stood surety for my treatment costs at Hershey. As a plan B, he had already lined up for my treatment by Dr. Willis of Pinnacle Health Center, Harrisburg, PA.

Mrs. Sarla Goel: She is a highly accomplished person. She is a lady of great personality, very humane, benevolent, and compassionate, with an understanding nature. She is included in every family matter. When I went to Hershey for chemo, she was in India. She gave us her entire house. We stayed there for about three months. After she returned to America, she provided me with full care and support. She also accompanied me to hospital visits on several occasions. I really value her support.

Dr. R.K. Ranga: He is my father's all-weather friend. He was in the hospital throughout my mother's illness. Mrs. Ranga always remained with my mom in the hospital. Whenever the family was facing a dilemma— whether it was my mom's surgery or my birth—he firmly stood by my father. We two families share a strong bond.

Dr. Sarla Malhotra and Dr. Bhushan Kumar: Dr. Sarla monitored my mother's treatment and was a strong motivation factor during her chemo. She took personal interest in my treatment and always remained available. More than a doctor, she is an aunt to me and my brothers.

A noble soul, Dr. Bhushan is beyond description. Though a skin specialist, he is a jack of all trades. He brings a smile to everyone's faces through his wit and humor. Dr. Bhushan and Dr. Sarla always encouraged my mother during her treatment. They made my life easy and continue to push me ahead in life. The couple is my first contact in emergency.

Dr. J.D. Wig: He is a doctor of high repute. After working with PGI Chandigarh for 35 years, he is currently a Senior Consultant at Fortis Hospital, Mohali. He is constantly surrounded by an aura of serenity and calmness. He operated on my mother in the year 1999 and, fourteen years later, he led the team of surgeons for my operation. His presence is a huge source of support for all his patients.

Dr. Nitya Nand: He is a Senior Professor of Medicines and Medical Superintendent at PGI Rohtak and an old family friend. I remember, even as a child, whenever I had minor illnesses like a cough or cold, my father would instantly ring him, and he would give me the prescription via phone. He constantly stayed in touch with the family during my mother's illness as also during mine.

Ms. Seema Chettri: Seema came to stay with us sometime after my fifth birthday. She left for Connecticut to pursue her Master's degree in 2007. When my dad and I went to America for two years, Seema stayed with us. After completing her MS degree in 2010, she resumed her job at Chandigarh. We share a close bond.

The McClelland family: The entire family gives us a warm hug whenever we meet. Mr. Rob is a very gentle and kind person. He protected me like a guardian in 3rd and 4th grades. His wife, Mrs. Barbara, also possesses a great personality and makes me feel like home whenever I visit them in North Carolina. She also educates me on common day-to-day life etiquette. They sent me a care package at the time of my chemo. I extend my heartiest greetings to each member of the McClelland family.

Mr. Jugal Verma and Mrs. Dinesh Verma: Settled in Maryland, USA, the Vermas are very close to our family. Both the families stay in touch on regular basis. I was in perfect health when we visited them in June 2013. My cancer, diagnosed a couple of months later, was equally shocking for them. Immediately, they started coordinating with doctors in their circle. They even visited us in Hershey during my chemo. Dinesh aunty and I share a personal bond. She has also successfully battled cancer. From the start of my cancer journey, she has encouraged me greatly.

The Hershey team: I cherished my treatment at Hershey and greatly value their Medical team. On our very first visit to the Pediatric Cancer Care unit of Penn State Children's Hospital, Hershey, I was given a warm welcome. The place looked like a play school loaded with toys and balloons. The staff nurses wore colorful clothes. There was no usual hospital odor; on the contrary, the entire place was full of fragrances. My dad exclaimed that it was like a five-star hotel after they gave us a tour of the place. Dr Fecile was visibly pleased with the comments. The entire team was excellent throughout my treatment.

DPS Chandigarh: When we were looking for schools for my kindergarten admissions in 2004, the family decided DPS on the recommendation of Mr. Ram Singla. The then Principal, Ms. Sunita Tanwar, and my class teacher, Ms. Shruti, took personal care in my well-being. I was in US for 3rd and 4th grade. When I returned in 5th grade, the current Principal, Mrs. Reema Diwan, welcomed me back with her usual broad smile. The DPS support staff and faculty provided me full support during and after my entire illness. During my four months stay in US for chemotherapy, my teachers emailed me class notes. When I returned after chemo in January 2014, my 8th grade exams were drawing close. The school made sure I was free from exam fever. Despite four months' absence from school, I did not feel neglected or lagged behind. The school support continued unabatedly. My peer group is equally important in my life. Thank you DPS.

Chapter 1

My mother was diagnosed with carcinoma stomach in 1999, at the age of 39. For about a year prior to this diagnosis, she had been complaining of persistent stomach aches, but had not yet sought medical advice about what the cause of them might have been. My maternal grandfather, Dr. Parma Nand, was a doctor of repute in Patiala, Punjab. He was very famous and formed part of the "who's who" of Patiala. Though he mostly worked as an Ayurvedic doctor, being a graduate of Tibbia Medical College in Delhi, he also practiced allopathy (the treatment of diseases with drugs designed to counteract the symptoms, and what most people would think of as standard medical practice) and performed surgeries in his private clinic. He immediately decided to oversee my mother's treatment.

For Western readers who might not be familiar with the term, Ayurvedic medicine is a traditional approach to healing that focuses on finding a balance between the body, mind, and spirit. In some countries, it is considered a form of alternative medicine, aimed at overall wellness than it is designed to fight disease. In India, however, where the practice got its start, it's more widely accepted as a potential treatment for a wide range of ailments. My mother certainly had full faith in my grandfather's methods, having seen him practice medicine throughout her life. Even though she trusted his approach, after about a year of the treatments overseen by my grandfather there was a drastic shift in my mom's health. Her appetite diminished drastically, and she started to lose weight.

During the years leading up to this, throughout 1997 and 1998, my father had mostly remained out of town. His job demanded that he travel often. He was an attorney by profession, maintaining a law office in Anand Niketan, New Delhi. For the preceding ten years, he had also worked as the official spokesperson and legal adviser of Jharkhand Mukti Morcha (JMM), a political party whose main focus was spearheading the movement for a separate Jharkhand State. They would achieve this goal a few short years later, in November of 2000, the fruition of a movement that had started nearly a century before. At that time, though, Jharkhand was a part of Bihar State, in North -east India—over 1,000 miles from the city of Chandigarh, in northern India, where my family lived—and while working for JMM, my father used to regularly visit far off places in Jharkhand areas of Bihar State.

When my father would return to Chandigarh, he would know of my mother's occasional stomach pain and the treatment she was being given by her father, but he wasn't there to see its progression day by day. When he returned home in the summer of 1999, then, the sudden change in my mother's condition was very pronounced. He was alarmed by the speed and extent of her weight loss and insisted that she received medical check-ups from qualified doctors in more modern medical practices. He also persuaded my grandfather to consult specialists. He took my mother for a consultation with a renowned Gastroenterologist in Patiala, who later performed endoscopy that confirmed my father's worst suspicions: all was not well in her stomach.

My parents had met when they were in their early twenties and had enjoyed a blessed and happy life up to this point. Their marriage was arranged, at the suggestion of my maternal grandfather, Dr. Parma Nand. The idea of arranged marriages has a certain stigma in Western nations, but in India they remain a natural part of the social and cultural landscape. They are not the forced unions between unwitting participants that an American reader might presume; rarely are marriages arranged for children, anymore, and both partners typically have at least some say in whether or not they want to wed. Both my parents had already started their adult lives before the marriage was suggested. My mother had recently graduated from college, earning two degrees (a BS in Science and a BS in Education). My father was at a similar point in his own life, having just started practicing law a couple of years before. Even though he was relatively new to his career, though, he'd already made something of a name for himself as an aggressive litigator. Some of his cases had even earned national attention, with stories about them published in national newspapers.

It was my father's work as a litigator that brought him initially to my grandfather's attention. He'd visited my father in Chandigarh in this professional capacity, a matter related to a pending litigation being handled by my father's firm. I don't believe my grandfather had any intentions to find his daughter a husband when he made the trip. After they spoke, though, he was impressed by my father's work ethic, intelligence, and bearing—things that would make him an excellent match for my mother. Marriage was the next major upcoming milestone in my mother's life, now that she had completed her education, and after some discussion the union was arranged. By August of 1981, my parents were married.

It is typical in India for the wife to adapt to the lifestyle of her husband and focus primarily on the home and family, rather than a career. This isn't always the case, of course—and wasn't always the case in the early

1980s when my parents married—but is typically the way things go. My mom had applied for a post as a science teacher prior to the arrangement of her marriage, and a few days after the ceremony she received an appointment in a government school. After some discussion, though, my father persuaded her not to take the job and to instead live with him to Chandigarh, where she could focus on raising their family. She was one of the best-educated full-time homemakers in their entire neighborhood.

My mother and father had very different upbringings and childhoods. My father had grown up in a working class family and was accustomed to working hard to get the things that he wanted—he had no trouble working even a 20-hour a day schedule without losing his focus, and it was this dedication and willingness to put in the time and effort that had gotten him to where he was, practicing law in a major city. My mother, on the other hand, was from a comparatively wealthy background. Her father's fame and stature as a doctor in Patiala had given the entire family this kind of privileged status—and it was a large family, too. My mom was the sixth of seven children, and as she'd grown up her family had only grown, as three of her brothers got married, had children and started families of their own. She was the kind of woman who thrived in this large family environment, making many happy memories with her family back home before she grew up and moved on into her own adult life.

These differing upbringings did give my parents a different perspective, and this stuck with them in many ways as they respectively entered adulthood. My mother had an appreciation for the finer things in life, for example. She loved both cooking and eating good food, for example, a trait she would end up passing along to both my brothers and myself. My father was more practical in this regard, seeing food as necessary sustenance for survival rather than something to be savored and enjoyed. In other ways, though, they were similar. My mother was a perfectionist, very willing to work hard to make things exactly right; in this regard, his strong work ethic and her drive for perfection meshed together well.

My parents didn't have completely different upbringings, though. Just like my mother's family, my father's family was also on the larger side. Several of his siblings lived with him when he and my mom were married, including his mother, three younger brothers, and two of his older sister's children, since she had remarried after divorcing their father. This meant that my mom looked after a family of seven as soon as she moved in with my father in Chandigarh—something that probably felt very familiar to her, after having grown up with as many siblings as she did. She bonded quickly and easily with my dad's family, caring for them as if they were her own family and earning their love and respect in just a short period of time.

Soon enough, my parents started a family of their own. My oldest brother, Abhishek, was born in 1982, only a year after my parents were married. My other brother, Abhinav, followed five years later, in 1987. The family built a very nice life for themselves in Chandigarh, which at the time was about a tenth the size it is today—around 100,000 people, compared to the million plus that number in the city's population today. With my father's income as a lawyer and my mother at home to take care of the children, they had a comfortable upper middle-class lifestyle, and were rich in love—between my mother's side and my father's side, there were more than a hundred different families they could spend time with or call on in times of trouble. Even though my dad had to travel so much for his work, he would manage to work in a few hours at a time, three to four times a month, to spend some time with his sons or go out to a nice dinner and a movie with his wife. They were a happy couple, and as my brothers came along became a happy family.

By the time my mother started to have stomach pain, in around 1997, Abhishek was already in high school and Abhinav was in middle school. Both of them were very devoted to our mother and took care of her. She was there for whatever they needed, every minute of the day, providing emotional strength along with the basic needs. Throughout their school lives, neither of my brothers missed even a single day of school, both of them earning 100% attendance certificates upon their respective graduation. They never have any problem with discipline or paying attention to school—by all accounts, they were perfect students with excellent character, very respectful, honest, and responsible, serving as role models for their peers in school. Abhishek especially was something of a carbon copy of our mother: pleasant, helpful and a bit of an introvert. Abhinav was more of a mix of both parents in terms of his personality and was a bit more of an extrovert personality than our older brother, but he, too, bore the definite imprint of our mother's care and attention.

My mother had poured her entire self into raising her sons, and it definitely showed in how they conducted themselves, even as children. Her compassion and dedication were a source of strength for the entire family, and while I wasn't yet born—or even yet a thought—when she was diagnosed with cancer that first time, I can only imagine the fear and helplessness my brothers and father felt when they saw her health begin to fail.

After the Gastroenterologist in Patiala saw the initial results from the endoscopy, he advised my father to get a second opinion from another Gastroenterologist closer to home, in Chandigarh. My father consulted with Dr. M. L. Sarwal, a Gastroenterologist who had a private clinic in the city. Dr. Sarwal performed another endoscopy before he made any further decisions about my mother's treatment. This test report confirmed the worst-case scenario; my mother had cancer in her stomach.

Before she'd started to complain of stomach pains a few years prior, my mother had shown none of the warning signs that would lead us to believe she'd developed cancer. Cancer in general is an illness that can be difficult to identify and diagnose, even by trained medical professionals. It is still this way today, and even less was understood about it in the late 1990s when my mom was diagnosed. Stomach cancer especially can be a troubling ailment to correctly diagnose and treat because so many of its main symptoms can be caused by a variety of other ailments. Appetite loss, unexpected weight loss, and persistent stomach pains are the most common indicators—ultimately, the symptoms that led to my mother's successful diagnosis—but these can also be caused by everything from ulcers to the flu virus. It's because of this that stomach cancer is often not diagnosed until fairly late in its progression.

It was good luck that my mother's diagnosis had come in time for a surgical solution, but looking back, it is possible that this solution was not reached soon enough. Only about one out of every five known occurrences of stomach cancer are diagnosed early enough to prevent it from spreading to other areas of the body; the remaining 80% of the time, the disease has advanced past the point of metastasis before noticeable symptoms begin to show. This is one of the reasons post-surgical treatments are considered so important for stomach cancer, especially. Removing the known tumor isn't always enough to also remove the disease.

My dad shared the distressing news with the Singla family, his closest friends and mentors in Patiala, as soon as the diagnosis had been confirmed. Ram Singla Uncle, who was around my father's age, had been someone my father could rely on in tough times since they were both young men, and after their respective marriages they remained very involved in each other's family lives. During the span of their friendship, my dad had also grown close to Uncle Ram's older brother, Mr. B.K. Singla, who immediately traveled from Patiala to Chandigarh and joined my father for a meeting with Dr. Bhushan Kumar and Dr. Sarla Malhotra, the doctors who would be establishing my mother's treatment plan.

Dr. Bhushan and Dr. Sarla were senior doctors working at the Postgraduate Institute of Medical Education and Research (PGIMER) in Chandigarh. As a research institution as well as a medical hospital, PGI was the best place to go in the whole of North India to get access to the most modern and advanced cancer treatment methods. Dr. Sarla's main expertise was gynecology, and she was a senior professor in that field at PGI. Dr. Bhushan was Professor and Head of the Department of Dermatology at the institution. As impressive as his medical knowledge was, he was equally known for being a noble soul who could make anyone smile. They both had a strong social bond with our family. Of all the doctors in Chandigarh, my dad trusted Dr. Bhushan and Dr. Sarla the most. Both suggested consulting Dr. J. D. Wig, the head of the Gastroenterology department at PGI, to get the best treatment for my mother's condition. Dr. Bhushan fixed an appointment for consultation with Dr. Wig.

My mother was so beloved by her family and community that this meeting became something of a group affair. Not only did my grandfather join my dad and Mr. Singla for the meeting, my dad also called Dr. R.K. Ranga, an officer of the Indian Administrative Services (IAS) and a close friend of the family. During the meeting, my father was impressed, not only by Dr. Wig's expertise, but also by his personality. He exuded a sense of serenity and calmness that made everyone in the meeting feel instantly more at ease. Dr. Wig advised that my mother should go in for immediate surgery, a decision that Mr. Singla and Dr. Ranga fully supported. My grandfather, though, was firmly opposed to surgery. He insisted on continuing with her Ayurvedic treatment and spent a few days consulting with the specialists in his field. The news of my mother's diagnosis was shared with close family and friends. The Ayurveda doctors my grandfather had consulted with suggested some treatment options, including a cow urine treatment and a variety of home remedies, but they also told him my mother had less than a month to live. This was the main reason he was opposed to surgery; if she only had a few short days left, he didn't want her to spend it in the hospital in pain.

Dr. Wig understood my grandfather's concerns, but he also wasn't willing to concede that my mother was beyond help. He was finally able to convince my grandfather to agree to surgery by suggesting he perform it only after the number of days my mother was supposed to live according to the Ayurveda doctors. He further assured my grandfather that he would bring her back alive from the operating table, and that she would be in a much better shape after surgery than she was at the moment. On the assurances of Dr. Bhushan, Dr. Sarla, Dr. Wig, Mr. Singla and Dr. Ranga, my mother, who was otherwise very reluctant, gave her consent for surgery about twenty days later—well after the time table of when the Ayurveda doctors had said she would die. The next day, she was admitted to a private room at the PGI.

My father decided to put his work at the law firm on an indefinite hiatus so that he could devote his full attention to caring for the family, which at the time consisted of my mother and my two older brothers. My dad didn't want their lives to be impacted more than they had to be by their mom's illness and did everything he could to fulfill all of their needs. By this point, it was August of 1999. Abhishek was in 12th grade, preparing to pursue engineering in college, studying hard for his SAT and TOEFL exams; he had earned a name in his school as one of its smartest students, maintaining his perfect attendance and high marks despite the uncertainty of my mom's cancer diagnosis and treatment. Abhinav was in 7th grade at the time, and like

Abhishek consistently ranked at the top of his class. Both my brothers were studying at Yadvindra Public School (Y.P.S) in Mohali, one of the top private schools in the entire country of India.

Mr. Ramendra Jakhu, one of my father's friends, advised sending Abhishek to the United States for college. His son Vilakshan, who was one year older than Abhishek, had recently been admitted to North Carolina State University. When it came time for Abhishek to take his SAT and TOEFL exams, he scored a very high rank—high enough that he was admitted to more than a dozen universities in USA. In the fall of 2000, Abhishek joined the undergraduate class of the School of Electrical and Computer Engineering at the University of Maryland, College Park.

While my father saw to ensuring his sons work toward a bright future, my mother continued her treatments. She received the best possible care and attention from the medical staff at PGI, but they weren't the only ones there to support her. The many relatives and friends who had benefitted from her compassionate soul and emotional strength now turned up in droves to make sure she felt their love during this trying part of her life. Dr. Bhushan, Dr. Sarla, and Dr. R.K. Ranga were regular visitors. Mrs. Natasha Ranga, Dr. R.K. Ranga's wife, would sit by her side almost the whole day to keep her company. Of course, we had support from the entire Singla family, as well. Also, my father's closest friend, Mr. Ram Singla was always around and took over virtually all of the arrangements so my father wouldn't have to think about them. My grandparents had come from Patiala and decided to stay in Chandigarh for the entire duration of my mother's illness; my maternal uncle even brought along a number of blood donors. As perhaps could be expected, the entire clan kept visiting PGI despite restraints and requests for restricting visitors to prevent any sort of infection. These were by no means fair-weather friends. Many of them would show up again to support her when her cancer returned three years later—and were even on hand a third time, when my own cancer developed in 2013.

The passion of Dr. Wig for his profession is beyond description. A deeply spiritual person, he is a savior for both his patients and their families. My mother was surprised when he visited her hospital bed in the morning of 15th August. This is a national holiday in India on account of the nation's Independence, and many doctors would choose to spend it at home with their families instead of at work—but not Dr. Wig. On regular workdays, he would make it a point to visit all his patients at least twice a day. He was a constant source of positive energy, always with a broad smile on his face that would inevitably cheer up everybody around him. My mother developed complete faith in Dr. Wig over the course of her treatment.

Finally, my mother was relieved of the turmoil going on in her mind about the dangers of invasive procedures. She was still nervous, of course, but was at least not afraid to move forward with the treatment. As she was too weak for surgery at the time, she had been admitted in PGI undergoing tests and routine procedures for more than three weeks, longer than the number of days she was supposed to live as per the Ayurveda doctors who'd spoken to my grandfather. Dr. Wig was preparing her for surgery not only psychologically but also physiologically.

The day of the surgery was finally scheduled for a morning in late August. The procedure lasted for nearly eight hours. Mr. Singla and Dr. Ranga stayed with my father outside the operating room for its entire duration. Only when my mom was allowed to meet the family on her way out of the operating room, still lying on her stretcher in a semi-conscious state, did they heave a sigh of relief. Later in the evening, she was shifted back to her room to commence her recovery. While it had been long, the procedure was completely successful, and had gone as well as anyone could have hoped. The doctors had removed a large tumor from her abdomen and sent it along to the pathology department at PGI for testing, where the malignancy was confirmed.

After the surgery, my mother was kept at PGI for observation and to regain some of her strength. She was discharged from the hospital after two weeks. After surgery, my mother completely regained her health. She had no more complaints of stomach pains, and her appetite came back to normal. Dr. Bhushan and Dr. Sarla would visit her regularly, gently reminding her of the need for post-surgery chemotherapy and radiotherapy treatments, even if she was feeling as though she was back to full health. They had been advised by the oncology department of PGI to persuade her into receiving this further treatment, a necessary step to reduce the risk of disease recurrence in the future. Like all cancer patients, my mother was extremely apprehensive about the chemo and radiation. She had heard stories of pain suffered during chemo and while she wasn't vain, she wasn't looking forward to the hair loss, either.

One of my father's friends, visiting from Denver, USA, took my mother's pathology report for consultation with the doctors there. These American doctors commented that my mother's tumor was extremely mild and doubted whether it had in fact been malignant at all. Since my mother was already apprehensive about undergoing further treatment, she took this as proof that she didn't need chemotherapy, and become more resistant to the idea that she truly needed to go through the potential horrors of these very intense procedures.

Ultimately, it was Dr. Sarla who convinced her that follow-up treatments were, in fact, necessary to ensure her continued health. My father accompanied her to the treatments: six three-day cycles with a gap of 21 days in between them, a nine-day drug regimen, and six radiotherapy sessions with the whole treatment lasting about five months in total. Dr. Sarla and Dr. Bhushan monitored my mother closely throughout, giving her encouragement and motivation to keep pushing forward.

Meanwhile, the eradication of the cancer in her stomach wasn't the only change going on in my mother's life and body. I was conceived during this time span while the radiotherapy treatments were still going on, though they didn't realize what had happened at first. I was visible on the ultrasound reports taken by the doctors at PGI in the spring of 2000, but I was still small enough at that time that they didn't realize I was a separate mass. They thought I was simply a part of the tumor. It wasn't until after the treatments had concluded the summer of that year that they realized the lump they'd seen was a fetus.

Though I hadn't yet been conceived until near the end of my mother's first battle with cancer, I have since heard many stories of how my family endured. My father made a point of making my brothers his first priority, keeping them on track with their education but also paying close attention to their emotional well-being. He used the large amount of social capital he'd accumulated over the course of his career to secure the help my mom needed to manage her illness. He would do the same when my mother's cancer returned, and again when I was diagnosed with cancer 13 years later. He had always been the strong foundation of our family, providing for our financial needs, and now he stepped up to fill new roles when he was most needed.

My mom lost her hair completely, as is usual after chemo. My father contacted a friend of his in Calcutta, S. Sunder Singh, who was a very senior police officer (IPS) posted in West Bengal. He arranged for some wigs to be sent to her. As it turned out, though, she barely had to use them. Her hair grew back faster than usual; before much time had passed at all, she had a full head of beautiful hair, even thicker and healthier than it had been before her illness. As the days passed, it certainly seemed as though the danger had passed. She was happy, healthy, and alive, having won her battle against cancer.

My mother was an extraordinary human, and no one knew it better than her friends and family. My grandfather, aunts, and uncles had known of her incredible kindness and strength of character since she was little; my father's family had come to regard her with a deep love and respect in the years since their marriage, coming to see her as a role model for both her sharp intelligence and her open heart. When friends and family heard of the success of her treatments, there was much celebration in both Chandigarh and Patiala. Her good nature was renowned along with good reason—and her friends and family were happy at the thought of being able to put this struggle in the past. There was no way to know, of course, that this was only the beginning of the family's fight against cancer—a fight that would span decades and generations before it was vanquished completely.

Chapter 2

My conception in early 2000 was about as unusual as it could be. Like I mentioned before, the doctors didn't even realize initially that I existed. My mother was still undergoing post-surgery chemo and radiation therapy in January 2000 when I was conceived; nobody expected my coming. The regular ultrasound proved deceptive, and the lump that appeared during the scan was misinterpreted as a side effect of my mom's surgery and continuing treatment. My existence, in fetus form, remained hidden from the medical world until July, when my mother was in the beginning of the seventh month of her pregnancy.

There were mixed reactions among family members to the news of my conception. The doctors were shocked, not just because of the post-cancer treatment she was still undergoing but also because of my mother's age. They were skeptical that I would survive to term and concerned that I wouldn't be born healthy even if I did. The ultrasound reports taken at PGI in July showed evidence of potential deformations (like not having a leg, an arm, or being mentally challenged), something that wasn't uncommon among children conceived during radiation therapy, and that was also more likely among older mothers.

My maternal grandfather shared the concerns of the doctors. He had seen children born sickly or with handicaps after having been conceived while the mother was undergoing intense medical treatments. What was worse in his mind was the potential risk to my mother's health that could come as a result of these health issues. He hadn't met me yet, after all; he was primarily concerned for the well-being of his daughter, my mother, especially after the year she had just endured. The added strain of creating a new life, he worried, could be too much on her recovery system. He was concerned about her emotional health, too, and the toll that it would take to lose a child after having already suffered such a stressful span of time. He strongly supported the views of doctors at PGI: abortion would be the best course of action.

Despite these concerns, my parents' reaction to the news of my impending birth was one of joy. For them, my conception was a gift sent straight from God—a long-awaited wish fulfilled. It seemed miraculous, given the unusual circumstances. My mother especially wanted me to be born and didn't want to destroy the fetus. If there was any chance at all of me being born healthy, that was a chance that she was determined to take. She was ready to welcome me into this world, whatever may come as a result of that decision.

My mother confided this desire of hers to my dad and my parents together consulted Dr. Sarla Malhotra, the head of the Gynaecology Department at Government Medical College and Hospital in Chandigarh. Dr. Sarla was the first person from the medical profession who was staunchly opposed to the idea of abortion. She understood and sympathized with my mom's desire to keep me, her miracle daughter. It was heartening for them to have finally found some support from the medical community, but the advice of the doctors was still overwhelmingly in favor of abortion. Even my grandfather seemed to have no hope that I would be born whole, despite knowing my mother's strong feelings on the matter.

For some time, my parents had both been regular visitors to a holy man by the name of Pinjorewale Babaji, who lived in a nearby village called Pinjore. My father decided to go see him in August in order to seek his advice on whether they should follow my mother's wishes, allowing me to be born, or go with the advice of the doctors and my grandfather, who believed the fetus should be destroyed. My father didn't undertake this journey alone. Mr. B.K. Singla and Mr. R.K. Ranga accompanied him, standing by his side and providing moral support just like they had been doing for the entirety of my mother's illness.

Not wanting to ask his advice without being able to offer any notes or information for him to review, they took a bag full of my mother's medical records with them. When Babaji saw them arriving with their bag of medical records, though, he told them to keep the bag away. Before they explained a single thing about our situation to him, Babaji firmly announced that my mother should allow her baby to be born. Furthermore, he predicted that she was going to give birth to a baby girl. This little girl—me—would not only be born healthy, Babaji said, but her birth would be a boon for my mother's health, restoring her to the way she'd been before the cancer struck.

Babaji further instructed my father that the baby should be named after the Hindu goddess Durga. This mythological figure from the Hindu pantheon is often depicted as a fierce warrior—a fighter against evil, defender of the good, and slayer of demons. This was an auspicious name to be chosen for a female child, since she is generally seen to represent the power of the feminine energy, and is one of the most prominent goddesses in the entirety of the Hindu religion.

My dad and his friends were overjoyed at hearing this positive prediction from the holy man. They rushed back to Chandigarh to share the good news with my mom and tell her the instructions Babaji had given them about how I should be named. Both my parents were excited on knowing that they would have a daughter, after two sons. Another spiritual figure had previously told my parents that if they should have a daughter, her name should begin with the letter "A." They spent the next few days searching through the many synonyms for Durga, eventually stumbling across the name "Aditi" on the list. This would fulfill both of my naming requirements. All that was left for them to do now was wait until my birth, to see if Pinjorewale Babaji's prediction had been true.

On September 26, 2000, the due date of my arrival, the doctors told my father to go attend his court work as usual, and that he should be mentally prepared to take away my dead body at 2pm. At around 2, my father reached the hospital in his lawyer's dress—a black coat and white trousers—knowing that I would be born healthy despite the warning. Babaji had told him as much, and my father had full faith in him. He was still overjoyed to see me when the nurse pulled me out of the incubator. He held me up in the air made me swing up and down like a toy. I was a few weeks premature, and as a result of this I was a tiny, underweight baby—only two and a half pounds on the day of my birth. He says that I was like a chuhiya, a small mouse, that could fit in his blazer pocket. I refused to accept this statement until Dr. Sarla confirmed it was true. Aside from this minor issue, though, I was healthy and normal, all vitals intact, with no deformities or apparent problems as a result of my mother's cancer treatments. My grandfather—who had continued to doubt whether I could be born healthy, unconvinced by the holy man's prediction—refused to believe that I was truly whole and healthy until he examined me himself. He looked me over from head to feet, counting each of my fingers and my toes, confirming that I had all my twenty digits. Finally he had no choice but to admit I was a normal baby girl. As far as he was concerned, this was nothing short of a miracle.

My family has always been a close-knit clan, and my birth brought smiles and good cheer to everyone within it. My parents immediately called Sonu Bhaiya in America and gave him the good news. Abbu Bhaiya was, of course, there with them in the hospital and one of the first people to help welcome me into the world. That day, dad distributed sweets to the whole hospital staff, the entire neighbourhood and all his friends at the court (around 100 people). There were grand celebrations over the course of the next few days as news of my healthy birth spread through my relatives, especially once my mom and I had both received clean bills of health and were cleared to go home from the hospital. A few days after I went home, Pinjorewale Babaji—who rarely paid anyone a visit to their home—came to see my parents and bless the newly born child.

By the time my first birthday rolled around, my mother's cancer was still in remission; Babaji's prediction that my birth would prove a good omen for my mother's health seemed as though it had been accurate. As small as I had been when I was born, I was now growing at a normal rate, although I was still on the small side for a child my age. It at least seemed as though my family had finally passed through its trials.

My parents threw my first birthday celebration in the Officer's Mess of Punjab Police. Neither of my brothers had ever been given a birthday party with as much pomp and show involved as the one my parents threw for me in 2001—and with me too still young to even remember it. The party wasn't really for me, though, I realize looking back. It was a celebration of everything my family had endured since my mother was first diagnosed with cancer, a chance for us to have fun together and gather for something purely positive. Almost everyone was there—my mom's family, my dad's family, and all of the family's closest friends, around 300 well-wishers. From what I understand, it was quite the party.

I was too young when my mother was still alive to have many memories of her, but I do remember her dropping me off at play school, Ashiana, when I was around three years old. There were times I didn't want her to leave me there alone. I would cling to her clothes when she tried to drop me off in the morning, and I always rushed out to meet her when she came to pick me up a few hours later.

I also know that I was sitting on my mother's lap the first time I received a blessing from Swami Debananda ji, although I was too young still at that point in time to remember the occasion. Swamiji is a saint in the Vedic order who keeps his main ashram at Burdwan in West Bengal. This ashram is a place of much peace and beauty, situated across the street from an idyllic lake—exactly the kind of place that encourages visitors to undergo spiritual reflection and feel a deep sense of inner calm. Peace and self-reflection are two virtues that Swamiji has always made a point of instilling in his followers. My parents occasionally traveled to his ashram to hear his teachings, both before and after I was born. Every visit to Swamiji's ashram is a unique experience, one that always offers an opportunity for some new kind of spiritual development. While I may not remember my first visit to see Swamiji, it certainly made an impression on me. Throughout my childhood, any time I was feeling frustrated or upset I would ask my dad to call Swamiji. If I could even simply hear his voice on the other end of the phone, this would usually be enough to calm me down and make me feel better. My tears would magically roll up and a big smile would cover my face.

As few memories as I have of my mother from my early childhood, the exact opposite is true for the rest of my nuclear family. My father provided me with a strong, comforting presence from my very earliest memories onward, a constant that I was grateful to have in my life. He was so involved that I don't even remember feeling the absence of my mother. I had never truly known what it was like to live in a household with two parents; I only knew my dad would always be there when I asked for him, always watching over me and providing for my every need.

I have equally powerful memories of my brothers from when I was very young. Both of them are a lot older than I am; Abhinav was in 8th grade when I was born, and Abhishek had just started college. This age difference never mattered the entire time I was growing up, though. It often meant we were physically far apart, but our emotional connection was strong throughout my life. If anything, it simply meant they treated me more like a daughter than a sister.

As soon as I could talk, I started calling my brothers by their nicknames: Sonu Bhaiya for Abhishek, and Abbu Bhaiya for Abhinav. These nicknames stuck; to this day, I very rarely call them by their full names. Sonu Bhaiya is a towering presence in all of my early memories; I could always feel him standing with me, even when he was far away. Abbu Bhaiya was my close companion for my early years, helping my dad to care for me and watch over me, until he too moved to the United States to obtain his college education starting Fall 2005.

Although I didn't know my mother's personality for my part, I am told my two brothers both have qualities that reflect her strong influence over their early life. This makes sense, of course; she had raised them full-time while my father was frequently away on work, so she was the main person who was around to emulate when they were children. Like many siblings, they are similar in many respects but quite different from each other in others. Sonu Bhaiya is a very straight-forward and single-minded person. He likes to get things done in a very orderly manner, preferring not to waste time. At the same time, though, he's also very gentle and compassionate, and that was the side of him I saw the most often when I was little. He's also an extremely organized and clean person. Many of these characteristics are ones he picked up from our mother, and of the three of us, my father tells me he's the most like she was.

Abbu Bhaiya, on the other hand, is a more even mix of both our parents' qualities. He's caring and helpful, like my mother was. When I started going to school, he would take care of everything the night before— preparing my uniform by washing it, ironing it, and laying it out on my bed; filling my lunchbox with a different, unique meal every day; even waking me up and helping me to get clean and fed. As long as I can remember he has been very protective of me. Along with his caretaker instincts, he shares my father's love of socializing. He's always been popular and had lots of friends at every school he's attended.

After my mom's first round of cancer treatments ended and she was declared to be in remission, Sonu Bhaiya left for the United States and was enrolled at the University of Maryland as an undergrad freshman. My dad visited Sonu Bhaiya in December 2000 and took pictures of me to him. This was the first time Sonu Bhaiya saw my photos.

When I was around three years old, in the summer of 2003, my parents decided to take me and my brother to Maryland for a visit. We hadn't had many opportunities to be together as a family since Abhishek had started his studies, so my parents decided to make the most of this one, arranging for us to stay in the United States for a full two months.

At the time of our visit, Sonu Bhaiya was sharing a two-bedroom apartment near the University of Maryland campus in College Park, Maryland. We stayed there with him over the summer. College Park was a smaller town, but it wasn't a very far drive from the nation's capital, Washington DC, so we had plenty of things to do while we were there. Abhishek had a car and he'd use it to take us to different places around the city.

I was still very young, of course, and I don't remember this trip, but looking at the pictures I can well imagine the joyful days I spent with my brothers and my parents, and the fun that we all had. We went to summer carnivals, took rides around the countryside, and visited the big tourist sites, like the Washington Monument. Sonu Bhaiya had always focused on developing my mind, so I'm sure he showed me lots of exciting and interesting things along the way.

The trip wasn't just about seeing the sights. We also had a lot of friends in the United States, and my parents made a point of visiting as many of them as we could during our time in the country. This included the family of Mr. Jugal Verma. They were living in Maryland, so it was an easy matter to pay them a visit during our trip. We also paid a visit to Dr. Ram Goel, in Camp Hill, PA, the family friend who'd helped convince my mom to send Abhishek to America for college. The United States was on the other side of the world from our home, but the number of friends we had there certainly made it feel a lot closer.

In the photos from this trip, my mother is enjoying herself as much as the rest of us. She looks healthy, her hair thick and lustrous, a perpetual smile on her face. There were no signs of the cancer that would return in just a few short months.

For three whole years, from the summer of 2000 until the end of 2003, my mother had been completely healthy. From what I've been told by my father and other close family friends, she had all but forgotten her cancer completely during this time. Some of the doctors she spoke to even suggested the tumor they'd removed may have been benign after all, supporting the mildness of it that had been noted by the American doctors when she was getting her initial diagnoses. Then, she was so sure she didn't have cancer that she didn't take care of her health. She went on eating street food, fried foods, etc. as she wished. Just as Pinjorewale Babaji had promised, my birth seemed to have restored her health completely. Within a year of returning to India after our 2003 vacation in the United States, though, two tragedies would strike our family: the death of my grandfather, and the return of my mother's cancer.

My maternal grandfather was a very jovial person. During the years of my parents' marriage, he had formed a close bond with my father. He'd gotten into the habit of coming to stay with my family, sometimes for a few weeks at a time. I've been told he was always overjoyed to see me. He would take me up in his arms with a big grin on his face, so thrilled to be spending time with his granddaughter. Unfortunately, I don't remember much about him; he passed away in December 2003. After that I became very close to my grandmother, who would be there through all the trials of my life until she, too, left her body in 2015 due to old age. While my grandfather was alive, he always kept his eye on my mother's health when he came by for these visits, but there was never any reason for alarm.

A few months after my grandfather died, in March of 2004, my mother started to experience severe stomach aches. Over the next few months she also lost her appetite and began to lose weight. These symptoms were similar to the ones she'd experienced prior to her first cancer diagnosis a few years erstwhile. My dad recognized this as a warning sign of something more serious going on and took my mom back to PGI to get a checkup and find out if she needed further treatment.

The results of these tests were not encouraging. She was diagnosed with blood cancer. Her white blood count had already fallen below the danger level. No one was quite sure what had caused the recurrence. Possibly her stomach cancer hadn't been completely eradicated by the chemo and radiation treatment, despite all indications that her system had been clear. Some of her doctors speculated there had been a lacuna in the post-surgery and post-chemo follow-up. Whatever the cause, this cancer was at a far more advanced stage than her stomach cancer had been a few years earlier, and the predictions of the doctors were far more grim.

I called Abhishek with the news, and he immediately made plans to return from the United States. He had intended to pursue his Master's degree at the University of Maryland in the coming Fall. Coming back to India now could potentially put those plans in jeopardy, but he didn't even hesitate before making his decision; he needed to be with the family.

My mother was admitted to PGI in April of 2004. Many of the staff members there knew her already—some because of the time she'd spent there during her first round of cancer treatments, others who were family friends from long before her first experiences in the hospital. One of these old friends was Dr. Nitya Nand, one of the senior professors at PGI Rohtak. He'd always been just a phone call away throughout my childhood whenever I had colds or other minor illnesses. Once my mother was admitted, he made a pointing of keeping close tabs on her progress, even though he wasn't the doctor directly in charge of her care. We knew that she would be in good hands while she was at PGI.

A few days after she was admitted, there was a steep drop in my mother's blood platelet levels. After reviewing her reports, and given this most recent development, the oncology department at PGI told my father they could provide no further treatment. They discharged her, advising us to take her home and make her comfortable, because they could not allow her to continue to stay in the hospital. In their eyes, she had no hope for recovery.

My father was not satisfied with this diagnosis. After all, my mother had beaten cancer once; with the strength of the family behind her, he knew she could do it again. He consulted with two doctors at Fortis Hospital in Mohali, one a surgeon by the name of Dr. Raina with whom he'd consulted previously, when my mother's health first began to decline again. The other was an oncologist named Dr. Rajiv. The infrastructure at Fortis Hospital had a five-star rating, far superior to any of the area's government hospitals, and their facilities boasted an ultra-clean environment and the most advanced technology available, although that meant expensive bills. The doctors at PGI were perhaps better experienced because of their clinical exposure, but the doctors at Fortis Hospital had access to more resources, and my father hoped this would help them find a treatment.

After reviewing her file, Dr. Raina and Dr. Rajiv admitted my mother to Fortis Hospital, assuring us of her recovery. The entire staff at Fortis was excellent while my mother was there. She felt downright pampered by the attentiveness of the doctors and ultra-modern environment. Even with the full benefits of medical science on our side, however, there was nothing that could be done. Her situation was worsening by the day. Watching her in the hospital was like seeing an open dance of death unfold before our very eyes. Soon, the day came that all of the doctors' best efforts resulted in no improvement. For all intents and purposes, Fortis Hospital had simply become a nursing home.

Hope was waning, but my father wasn't prepared to give up just yet. He spoke with Justice Amarjeet Chaudhary, a family friend, who suggested he should consult with Dr. B.D. Gupta. Dr. Gupta was the former head of the oncology department at PGI. Since leaving that institution, he'd started his own medical charity clinic in Chandigarh. My father reached out to him and explained the situation. Dr. Gupta made no assurances about what he could accomplish, but he agreed to take over my mother's treatment.

There was no reason for my mother to stay at Fortis Hospital, considering there was nothing more that could be done for her there. On Dr. Gupta's suggestion, we converted a portion of the house into a nursing home-type area. Access to this zone of the home would be very limited, minimizing the risk of infection, and it would contain all of the equipment required for my mother's treatment. Construction began immediately; a large room was added on to the second story almost overnight. Any visitors would be kept on the ground floor, with entry to the second floor restricted to necessary personnel.

By the time my mother arrived home, she was suffering from severe body aches and had lost her appetite extensively. Her health seemed to be deteriorating further with each passing day. Having been failed by medical science, my father decided to seek out holy men. A Sikh priest from the Central Reserve Police Force recommended that we chant a shabd, or hymn out of the Gurbani, the Sikh holy book. Another holy man my father spoke with suggested we should raise black dogs in the house. My father and I traveled to Kasuali, which was about 40 kilometers from Chandigarh, to buy a breeding pair. They delivered eleven puppies; this seemed to be an auspicious sign. Another room was built, this one on the first floor, a large room with a terrace that could serve as an oversized kennel for the entire pack. Having been told by the medical professionals that there was no hope, we were left entirely at the mercy of fate. Although dad contacted holy men belonging to different religious beliefs, all had said that they received no message from God that my mother would recover. This further strengthened our fear of losing her.

A few days after the puppies were born, Dr. Gupta suggested moving my mother to a hospital in Mohali called Silver Oak Hospital. This facility employed Dr. Gupta as a visiting consultant, giving him access to the emergency facilities if they should prove to be necessary. For the first few days after the move to the new hospital, my mom's pain subsided slightly. We knew we shouldn't let this raise our hopes up too much, however. I remember my dad one day casually asking Abhishek what his expectations were for our mother's recovery.

"Every day she lives is a bonus," he replied, candidly. I could not yet take this kind of mindset about her illness. I had just reached the age that I could start to make sense of what was going on around me, and I was certainly not ready to lose my mother so soon, when I was just beginning to understand the world. I remember sitting in the backseat of my dad's car on the drive to Silver Oak Hospital for a visit, praying to god to please save my mother. I didn't want to let her go.

A few days before my mother's death, I began to have intuitions of her going away. I could tell that, just from looking at the faces of my father and brothers, they were sensing the end was near as well. Shifting my mother to Silver Oak had extended her life for a few days, but we were all beginning to feel what Abhishek had said aloud: each day she lived was a gift.

Dr. Bhushan visited the hospital on my mother's last day alive. It was a Sunday morning, the fourth of July 2004. He'd come to consult with Dr. Gupta about my mother's treatment, arranging for platelets from PGI. Before they could discuss anything, however, my mother breathed her last in my father's lap. Even if we'd had the sense this would be coming, nothing could truly prepare us for her loss. I clung to the comfort of my father and brothers, and they to me and each other; together, we would find the strength to push forward.

Chapter 3

I was too young in July of 2004, when my mother died, to know what was going on at the house or sense the sadness in the air. I remember my family gathering all together, but at the time I didn't understand the reason for everyone being there. Mostly I was interested in playing with my cousins, some of whom I didn't often get to see, more than I was in what the adults were doing. Looking back, I wonder if my dad isolated me from the sadness of the adults on purpose, hoping to spare me the pain of the moment.

My father has always been the emotional rock of our family. I cannot recall ever seeing him cry in front of me; even in the months after my mother's death, he grieved in private and put on a strong face when he was around me and my brothers. He did everything in his power to keep me from being affected by the loss of my mother, even though that could not have been an easy time for him, either. My mother's death meant major changes would be happening in his life, beyond even the grief and emotional strain of losing someone so close to him. Before my mother's cancer, my parents had a very traditional marriage, as I mentioned earlier. My father worked full-time to support the family, while my mother stayed home full-time to take care of the house and kids. Because my dad's job required him to travel far and often, he wasn't very involved in the day to day care of either Abhishek or Abhinav when they were growing up, only seeing them for the occasional meal or weekend. Now, though, with my mother gone, both roles fell onto my father's shoulders.

We had helpers to take care of the household chores and prepare the family's meals. However, when it came to the work involved in raising me, my father did not delegate the tasks. He saw to my care personally, focusing fully on my needs. He had his law career to think about, too—there was still the need to earn money to keep us fed and healthy, and he maintained his office through my mom's illness and death—but he spent as much time as he was able to at home with me, even while he continued to look after things at his place of work.

My dad had a bit of extra help with me in that first year after my mother's death. Sonu Bhaiya had put his studies temporarily on hold and moved back to India when he heard of my mom's cancer. My mother died about four months after his return from the USA. Abbu Bhaiya was yet to prepare for his SAT, TOEFL, and other exams to apply to different schools for undergrad studies in the USA. This meant both of them were still around the family home while we all adjusted to life after my mother's death. Living under the same roof with both of my brothers was a new experience for me; even my earliest memories before this were from a time after Sonu Bhaiya had already left for the United States. With the large age difference between us, they sometimes felt more like extra parents than they did like brothers; they were certainly as devoted to me as a parent would be.

The fall after my mother's death, I reached the age that it was time for me to start school. Like many kids, I was both excited and nervous about this prospect. I liked playing with other kids but I was also still very shy at this point in my life, and the idea of meeting so many new people was a bit scary. My dad researched the options in the area and decided to send me to Delhi Public School (DPS) on the recommendation of his friend Mr. Ram Singla. The name of the institution is a bit deceptive. DPS is in fact a chain of private schools rather than a government-run institution, with branches located throughout India and beyond; they're well-known for the high level of education they provide. The branch in Chandigarh was fairly new when I was starting classes, having opened just in 2003, meaning the facilities in the school were all super-modern and in practically new condition.

Soon enough, we settled into a new routine. Every day, my dad would prepare food for me to take with me to lunch. He would also see to waking me up in the morning and making sure that I was dressed and ready to go in time. Sometimes he or one of my brothers would drive me all the way to school, but even on the days that I took the bus, whoever had dropped me off at the stop would stay there with me until they were sure I'd gotten onto the school bus safely. My class teacher, Ms. Shruti, took a personal interest in my well-being and kept a close watch over me during school to make sure that I was adjusting well. The DPS principal at the time, Ms. Sunita Tanwar, also went out of her way to make sure I felt welcomed at the school. It must have been a load off of my father's mind to know I would be in good hands after he'd sent me off for the day.

As enjoyable as the routine we'd fallen into was, we all knew it wouldn't be able to last forever. Abhishek's studies were set to resume in the fall of 2005, when he would start his work into earning a Master's degree at Southern Methodist University (SMU) in Dallas. Abhinav would also be going to the United States for that same term, though he would be starting his undergraduate studies in the School of Public Affairs at American University in Washington, DC—very close to where Abhishek had completed his bachelor's studies.

The thought of Sonu Bhaiya and Abbu Bhaiya continuing their schooling gave me very mixed emotions. I obviously wanted my brothers to pursue their education and secure themselves bright futures, but I also wasn't ready to say goodbye to them. It had been very nice having both of them with my dad and me the past few months; it would feel very empty once they departed for the United States.

In June and July of 2005, the summer before their respective semesters began, my father and I tagged along with Abhinav on a tour of the American University campus. This was mostly a practical trip, allowing Abhinav and my father a chance to see the campus in person, meet with some of the faculty members, and tour the facilities. We also visited a few apartments in the area, checking out potential places for Abhinav to live during his time at college. I rode around on my dad's shoulders during these visits, holding his bag with one hand while he kept my legs secure around his neck with the other.

In between taking care of these practical tasks, we snuck in some vacation time, too. We visited many of the same family friends we'd seen on our last trip to the United States. This time, though, I was old enough to remember the things we did and the people we saw. I started to form friendships of my own with the people my family was close to in the United States. These early visits were the start of life-long relationships with people near and dear to my family, many of whom would end up being invaluable help in the future, when I was undergoing my cancer treatment in America. Our trip in the summer of 2005 lasted a few weeks, if not as long as the trip the family had taken two years prior. It felt like it was over almost as soon as it started. Before I knew it, our time in the United States had come to an end and it was time for my father and me to return to India— without my brothers.

I had known the house would feel empty without my brothers around, but I didn't realize just how much I would miss them until they had actually departed from Chandigarh. It affected me much more when they left than it had when my mother died. Even though they were still alive, I had gotten so used to having them around all the time that their departure left a huge gap in my life. I couldn't cope with the vacuum left by both Abbu Bhaiya and Sonu Bhaiya moving away at the same time. I missed them especially when I returned from school each day. Before, one or both of them would be around when I got home each day, so I could tell them about my day. Sonu Bhaiya was always curious about how I was coming along in school and eager to help me develop my mind; I could always count on him to help me with my homework or quiz me about the things I'd been learning. If anything, I felt Abbu Bhaiya's absence even more keenly. He had been a constant presence in my life from my birth up to that point. With him gone, I couldn't help but feeling lonely.

I missed my brothers so badly that it started to affect my health. I had difficulty concentrating when I was at school, and sometimes couldn't do anything but stand in a corner and cry. I had the same class teacher that I'd had the previous year, Ms. Shruti, and she was still in the habit of keeping a close eye on me as she had my first year in the school. When she noticed how badly my brothers' departure was affecting me, she called my dad and reported to him about my declining emotional state. Even though my father was already very dedicated to making sure my needs were seen to, she suggested he take things a step further for a little while and do whatever he could think of to make me happy. She also suggested it might lift my spirits if I could see my brothers again, and that it might be a good idea to make plans for a visit.

My dad took this advice to heart. The first thing he did was to fill the refrigerator with all of my favorite treats: ice cream, chocolates, and cola, all of them at my own choosing. Once that was done, he took me to the travel agent's office and we finalized an itinerary to visit the United States in the winter. Now, instead of missing my brothers I could anticipate going to see them in a few months. This made a huge difference in my outlook, helping me get past the gap my brothers' absence had left in my life.

Finally, the day of our trip arrived. We planned to first travel to Washington, DC to visit Abhinav, then all three of us would go to Texas for a visit to Abhishek. On arriving in DC we went straight to Abhinav's apartment, where we would be staying while we were in the city. Between his studies, his work, and his new friends, he was leading a pretty busy life. Even though he was enjoying his time in DC, he missed me and my father terribly and longed to return to India. My dad convinced him that this homesickness was natural—this was, after all, the first time he had lived so far away from home, or on his own—but that it would likely pass as he settled into his routine at the university. It seemed that this trip wasn't only beneficial for my emotional health, but that it was a good chance for Abbu Bhaiya to see the people he'd been missing, too.

This was my first visit to the United States during the winter, and that meant a chance to experience wintery weather. For some people, this wouldn't have been a benefit, but for me seeing the snow fall was a great treat; it was something I didn't get to see very often. After Abbu Bhaiya's semester was over, we traveled together to Dallas to see Abhishek. There was no snow there, but it was the better half of the trip for me anyway—a chance for a few days of family togetherness.

Overall, it was a fantastic trip. I was sad when it was over, but I was still much happier when we went back to India in January of 2006 than I had been at the start of the year right after my brothers left. Even better, my father was already planning our next visit for the upcoming summer! I resumed my classes, counting the days until the start of summer vacation.

This trip to the United States that we took in the winter of 2005 ended up being the start of a long tradition. For the next three years, I visited the United States every summer and winter to see Sonu Bhaiya and Abbu Bhaiya, helping to make sure that none of us got too lonely without the others. Our relationship had always been strong, and if anything these experiences only made it stronger. We talked to each other regularly on the phone (Skype), but it was always very nice to get to see them face to face from time to time, too. No matter how often or how little we were able to be together, we never fought, even as I got older. In many ways, we had the perfect sibling relationships. Maybe this was part of why I always felt so much better whenever I could be around them.

My travels to the United States weren't just to see my brothers, either. Every year that I went I attended summer camp, as well. The first one, in the summer of 2005, was in Washington, DC. We'd picked it out partially because it was relatively close to Abhinav, which would make it easy for me to get to. I was five for this first summer camp. It was the first one I'd ever attended, and I had a whole ton of fun during my time there. At one point they took us to an aquarium, where we got to see all kinds of different sea creatures swimming around for us to observe. I learned a lot of new things about sea life that I'd never known before. We also watched movies together. The main one I remember us watching was *Ice Age*, which I loved because it was both really funny and had a great moral at the end.

The next two summers (2006 and 2007, when I was six and seven respectively) I went to a different summer camp. This one was in Harrisburg, Pennsylvania, which though it was in a different state wasn't too far from Washington, DC—only about a two and a half hour ride in the car. It was hosted by Harrisburg Academy, one of the top private schools in Pennsylvania. Their annual summer camp for kids my age was equally well-regarded. We found out about it through one of our close family friends in the United States, Dr. Ram Goel. Dr. Goel had opened his home to us every time we traveled through his area of the country, and had always been an excellent host. He had been a part of the governing body of the school and was friends with the principal of Harrisburg Academy, Dr. Newman, which was how he'd heard about the summer camp. Thinking I might be interested in attending, Dr. Goel introduced me to the camp's faculty, eventually arranging for me to attend.

As much fun as I'd had at the camp in DC, the one at Harrisburg Academy was even more exciting. Maybe the most unique thing we did during my time at the academy was that we went strawberry picking. The farm we visited to do this was about a twenty-minute drive from the camp itself. When we got there, the farm's staff handed each student a brown, rectangular basket and set us loose on the farm, where there were rows and rows of strawberries for us to pick. We had a whole hour to run around picking as many berries as we could from the various bushes, filling up our baskets until they were heavy with fruit and we couldn't put any more into them. Every day of the camp was another new, unique experience.

As much as I enjoyed the adventures we went on during these trips, I enjoyed being around the other kids even more. Like I've mentioned before, I was a pretty shy kid at this point, so getting to interact with so many new people in fun and different ways was a great thing for me. I not only learned a lot of things about the world around me, but I learned a variety of new social skills that helped me make more friends when I got back to school. It helped that most of the kids who attended these summer camps with me were like me. We were all the kind of kids who did what we were told and obeyed the rules and directions of the teacher. None of the kids were mean to me, and none of them were overly outspoken or too clever to the point that it felt intimidating to talk to them. In fact, I found that my fellow campers were generally very helpful, always willing to do what they could when someone around them was in need. I greatly enjoyed the summer camps and found them interesting all three summers that I went. I think every kid looks forward to summer vacation to some extent, if for no other reason than to have a break from classes, but I especially started looking forward to the season and the vacation to America I knew would come with it.

While my summer visits to the United States gave me something fun to look forward to during the school year, providing a nice distraction from the loneliness I felt after my brothers left, they couldn't change the fact that the house in Chandigarh still felt very empty with just my father and I living there. In May of 2006, some eighteen months after Abhishek and Abhinav moved to the United States, a new figure entered my life. Her name was Seema Chettri, and she'd moved from Sikkim to Chandigarh recently to start working for Spray Engineering Devices Limited, having recently graduated from Punjab Technical University with a degree in Chemical Engineering.

Seema was a young woman in her twenties when we met. She was very focused on her work. We'd go places together, developing the same tastes in food, activities, and clothes. Her job as a chemical engineer was in her field and with a good company, but she still planned to further her education. She started taking classes at a private institution called Grey Matter to prepare for the GRE and TOEFL exams. In the winter of 2007, she was admitted to a Master's program in Connecticut, pursuing a degree in Technology Management. She'd been living with me and my dad for long enough to become like an older sister to me. I was happy for her accomplishment.

In preparation for the start of her classes, the three of us—my father, Seema, and myself—took a trip to the United States in the last week of December 2007. Seema flew straight to Connecticut so she could start to prepare for her semester, but my dad and I decided to take a detour, taking advantage of the trip to see some family and friends as we'd done in the past. At this point, Abhinav was living in London, pursuing his studies at the London School of Economics (LSE). He'd arranged for me and my father to stay with him at the LSE residence hall during our visit, where we'd only be for a few days before continuing on to the United States.

Though we had only a short time in London, my memories from the visit stand out very vividly in my mind. It was a treat to stay on the LSE campus. I still remember the sumptuous breakfast they served, a spread with more variety than you'd find in most five-star hotels. My brothers had always taken great pleasure in showing me new attractions and delicacies, and this trip to London was no exception. It was wonderful to spend a few days with Abhinav, talking to him about his studies and his life in London, which was a fun new city to explore.

Abhinav wasn't the only one who'd moved on to a new home since the last time I had a chance to visit. Abhishek had finished his studies in Dallas by this point, and with his Master's degree under his belt was able to get a job with a company in Boston. This move ended up being really convenient for this current vacation because of all the friends and family members we had in nearby cities, like Harrisburg and Washington, DC. Boston was also conveniently located near Bridgeport, Connecticut, where Seema would be attending the university. For our nearly month-long vacation, we could make Boston our central location and from there easily get to everywhere else we wanted to go.

I visited quite a few new cities during this particular vacation. Boston and London were both busy, bustling cities that offered tons of things for us to do and see. The most unique of the new cities I visited on this trip, though, had to be Bridgeport, Seema's new home in Connecticut. Bridgeport is a sea-side city, the largest city in the relatively small state. It's located right at the mouth of the Pequannock River on Long Island Sound, in Fairfield County, a beautiful place though it was quite cold in the winter when we were visiting. While my dad and I were on our detour to visit my brothers in London and Boston, Seema had secured herself lodging for the upcoming school year, renting a spacious studio apartment on the campus of the University of Bridgeport where she'd be taking classes.

Since we would be bouncing around to different locations on this vacation more than we had on previous trips, my dad decided to rent a car to get us around. I would sit in a child's seat in the back and serve as the navigator, using a printed sheet of directions to get us to our various destinations. I took these navigator duties quite seriously, also being sure to monitor his speed and driving from my perch in the back seat—a habit I had gotten into on all of our road trips since I was about five. I loved long drives. Any time we stopped in a highway rest area, I would scour the brochures on display and pick up a few that looked like they'd be fun, paying special attention to any of them that were of particular interest to children. My dad would usually let me throw one of these new attractions onto our itinerary for the next day. This didn't always work out completely—I remember at least one time that the place I'd selected was meant more for children over the age of 12, and I couldn't do all of the fun things the park offered, but we still made the most of it, entertaining ourselves with the other activities that I could do at my age.

We of course stopped in and visited our friends in the Harrisburg, PA area while we were in the United States. Dr. Ram Goel was one of the people we visited. He had started teaching at Penn State University in Harrisburg, and the one who'd connected me with the faculty at Harrisburg Academy. His daughter, Sujata, is an accomplished dancer who has performed all over the world. She was an excellent teacher, eventually opening up her own dance academy in Harrisburg, which she continues to run to this day.

During that vacation in winter of 2007, we drove to visit Dr. Goel on a very snowy day. It was shortly after the Christmas holiday and the roads were empty of traffic, with no cars visible in any direction. My dad got distracted and crossed the yellow line. I shouted a warning, but it was too late; police were on our tail out of nowhere. We'd nearly reached the Penn State campus—it couldn't have been more than 100 feet away—so the police officer followed us the rest of the way to our destination rather than pulling us over.

I was so nervous that my dad was going to get in trouble, but the police officer turned out to be very friendly. Once he found out we were there to visit one of the professors on campus, he didn't even give my dad a ticket. He let us go with a warning once he'd finished his paperwork.

This small incident aside, our vacation was about as fun as it could be. As was often the case, I was a bit sad to be going back to India when it was over—now that Seema wasn't there anymore to keep me company. I was older now than I'd been when my brothers left, though, and I knew I would get to see them all again the next trip we took. I could always count on the friends we had in other places to take me on new adventures. My childhood travels taught me to focus on the positive, and while I still felt lonely from time to time, I always knew I would see them again if I could just be patient and wait for our next trip to come around.

Chapter 4

Between my brothers, Seema, and other family friends, I knew a lot of people who had moved from India to the United States by the time I was in elementary school. As many times as I had visited the country, though, I never thought about the possibility that I would live there myself until 2008, when my dad was appointed as an International Visiting Scholar, by the School of Law, University of North Carolina at Chapel Hill. The appointment was initially for one year, but this was extended for another one year after he was already there working.

In May of 2008, Seema was visiting my dad and me in India, having just finished her first semester as a Master's candidate at Bridgeport University in Connecticut. Following up on my father's upcoming appointment, she also started looking for schools in the Chapel Hill area, so the three of us could live together in the United States. She ended up securing a spot in a Master's program at North Carolina Central University's Department of Earth Sciences for the Fall term. NCCU was in Durham, less than a half-hour commute from UNC Law School, Chapel Hill where my father would work, and also from Creekside Elementary School, which I would be attending.

The three of us officially moved to North Carolina in August of 2008. I was about to enter the third grade; my father had enrolled me at Creekside Elementary School, which was only around five miles away from the Copper Ridge apartment complex where we had rented a three-bedroom apartment. The apartment complex was built right alongside a North Carolina state highway, which made it easy for us to get everywhere we needed to go.

A few days before my school year was set to start at Creekside, we had a visitor from India: Swami Debananda Ji, the founder of an Ashram in Burdwan, West Bengal. My father had been one of his disciples since I was very young. He and my mother had taken me to be blessed by him when I was a child, still too young to remember. On my first day of school my dad drove me, and Swami Debananda Ji accompanied us. The blessings he gave me on that day reassured me that my stay at the school would be memorable, enjoyable, and free of obstacles. Starting at a new school can be a nerve-wracking experience, especially for a kid as shy as I was, but the blessings given to me that day made me feel as though there was a layer of security around me. I knew I would face no difficulties and started my school year in peace and comfort.

Creekside Elementary was a public school. This was roughly equivalent to what was called a government school in India, at least in as much as it was operated by the state, although in terms of the building, infrastructure, and facilities like the library and cafeteria, it was far superior to government schools. It was even better than a lot of private schools in India in this regard, to be honest, at least the private schools I'd seen in Chandigarh—much too because there wasn't any uniform or strict dress code to follow.

Either my dad or Seema could have given me a ride to school every morning, and would have if I asked them to, but I liked riding the bus. My dad or Seema would accompany me from our apartment to the bus stop, which was still in the Copper Ridge complex but about a hundred or so yards from our front door. The bus supervisor, Mr. Rob McClelland, kept all the students in line and made sure that nobody was ever bullied during the ride. I didn't make any bus mates, preferring to sit quietly by myself during the ride, but nobody bothered me or made fun of me for it. Mr. Rob made sure of that. At the end of the school day, one of them was always waiting to pick me up when the bus dropped me off around two in the afternoon. The school had a policy that the bus wasn't allowed to leave a child at the stop unless someone was there to meet them. In the two years I attended Creekside Elementary, I never once had to wait for someone to come and pick me up. More often than not my dad was there waiting for me, but the few times he couldn't be, Seema was always there in his stead. Also, if all the seats in the bus were full, then another bus or van would come to pick up the student. No child would be made to stand or adjust in spaces, unlike the Indian buses (public transport and sometimes school ones too).

I loved going to school at Creekside Elementary. While many kids dreaded the school week and looked forward to their weekends, I was the opposite. When Sunday came, I always looked forward to Monday. It felt sometimes like spending time in a play school because of how many different things I learned all in one place. Everything about the school day was more fun and relaxed than I remembered it being in India. If the teachers had to discipline a student, they would always take them outside of the classroom to have a quiet discussion instead of scolding them in front of everyone. The teachers seemed to truly care about the well-being and development of their students, and it made the school a place that felt safe and comfortable.

The other students at Creekside Elementary were as welcoming and friendly as the teachers. Even though I was far from home, the atmosphere made it feel as though I was in my own hometown. I was pretty shy and didn't talk very much, but nobody ever made me feel like an outcast because of that or made fun of me for my introversion. There were students in the school from a lot of different cultures and backgrounds, so I didn't feel like I was an outsider just because I was born in another country. Some were from Vietnam, Mexico, or Spain, among other nations. I never experienced any racism, or felt at all lonely, rejected, or scared. If anything, the other kids were excited and curious about my different background. When lunch time came, students and teachers would sit and eat together in the same cafeteria. I would buy a drink, usually chocolate milk, but I often brought my own food from home, like parathas that my dad would make and pack for me. A lot of my friends at school hadn't seen them before. I explained that it was like stuffed bread and would let them share bites of it. We had a food festival at one point and my dad made halva, a sweet Indian dish that I knew my friends at school would love.

It didn't take long for me to settle into a routine. After school, I'd have a snack then settle in to do my homework while I watched something on TV, usually on the Disney channel, which played a lot of my favorite shows. The homework was easy, and there was a lot less of it than there was at schools in India. I usually finished it pretty quickly once I got home from school, especially if it was just a worksheet with some questions or math problems. Sometimes the homework we received also involved our parents, like watching or reading something together, or asking them to tell us a story.

Two times a week, a Spanish tutor, Ms. Fabiola, would come to the house. She was an excellent teacher, both making it very easy for me to learn how to speak and read this new language but also making it fun. We didn't just learn by memorizing words or by other boring, repetitive tasks. Sometimes she would bring Spanish story books that we would read together. Other times she would teach me Spanish songs, or we would watch videos in Spanish on YouTube. If there were any words I didn't recognize or understand, she'd stop and teach them to me. Every now and then she'd give me quizzes to test what all I'd learned. After Ms. Fabiola left, I would sometimes try to teach the words I'd learned to my dad, but he never seemed to pick up more than a couple words. I don't remember any Spanish words anymore, either. Mostly I just remember how exciting it was to study it.

The days that I didn't have my Spanish lessons I had lots of free time after I finished my homework. Sometimes Seema and I would go shopping together, usually at the South Point Mall although we also liked going to different places, too. A nice walk by the Jordan Lake was soothing when the wind blew. Other times we'd all go out to nice dinners at one of the restaurants affiliated with UNC. Our favorite ones to go to were the UNC Club, Chapel Hill and the Duke University Club. Not only was the food delicious, but I loved the fact that they kept a dish of candies sitting by the front doors. I'd usually sneak a few into my pockets as we were heading out the door at the end of dinner. Other times I'd go to UNC campus in the evenings. My dad and I often visited the Law School's library. They had a surprisingly extensive selection of popular movies on DVD which my dad would borrow for us to watch. My favorite movie at the time was *Legally Blonde*. They even had both sequels in their stock, and I must have borrowed them at least five times during the two years I spent in America, I loved them so much.

I had just as much fun in school as I did outside of it, though. Every single subject offered something new and exciting to learn. Art class was very different than it was in India. There, I thought art class was boring, but at my new school it quickly became one of my favorites. The teachers taught us both knife painting and brush painting and encouraged us to play with different techniques and approaches. I remember once I used a palette knife and a sponge brush to create a beautiful scenic landscape on a large sheet of paper. I used blue and white for the sky and waterfalls and made trees and bushes by putting brown on the palette knife then filling in the leaves with green and yellow on a sponge brush. It was an easy technique and the teacher taught it beautifully. This was so different than how things were taught in India. There, the teachers would often draw on the blackboard, or give the students a theme that they were supposed to create around, like underwater, scenery, flowers, or animals. Each student had a file where they would draw and color. In the art class at Creekside, though, the teacher went around the room and checked in with every student, guiding them step by step. I enjoyed the chance to show my creativity, eventually bringing one of the paintings home to show to my dad. I still have the landscape painting I did in that class.

I also looked forward to going to my music and drama classes. In the music class, we sang and learned how to play a lot of different instruments, including the piano, drums, and xylophone. What I really enjoyed most, though, were acting and dancing. I had taken dance classes back in India, but the kinds of dancing we did in school were very different. It was usually freestyle. We even put together plays that we performed on stage for our parents, teachers, and fellow students. In one play, I had the role of a mouse that chirped at a nest full of birds. Another time, at an assembly, we danced to a song from the *High School Musical* movie in front of the entire school. I was given a red t-shirt to wear for this, which had the number "3" printed on the front to show that I was in the third grade. This shirt is another memento I still have from my time at Creekside.

Of course, even though I liked school I was still a kid, and I really enjoyed the times we were able to be active, like gym class and recess. There was a playground where we would go for recess when the weather wasn't too cold. It had the usual swings and slide, and I would play on those sometimes, but I also liked just roaming around in the area outside, enjoying the windy weather. Gym class was where we'd have more organized physical activity. When you walked into the gymnasium at the school, you'd see markings on the floor and colorful sheets of paper attached to the walls, which together gave directions of diverse ways to get from end to end: hopping, running, jumping, jogging, skipping, or hula-hooping. Sometimes we'd play basketball or do exercises like push-ups. There was one time an expert at jumping rope who came to give a lecture and demonstrated a few tricks. I never would have thought the tricks he did were possible until I saw them with my own eyes. He moved with an incredible speed. It was a real treat getting to watch him and seeing what kind of tricks we could do with the jump ropes afterwards.

Even the more academic subjects that other kids might have thought were boring were interesting to me. This might have been because of the way I was brought up. Ever since I was old enough to remember, my brothers had taught me to love learning, encouraging me to ask questions and explore the world. I had grown up with the idea that it was fun to learn new things, and this attitude made it easy to fall in love with the many classes I attended during 3rd grade. In the social studies class, I learned about Rosa Parks, Nelson Mandela, and other leaders. It was interesting to read about the civil rights movement and anti-apartheid movement in the various parts of the world. I'd always enjoyed reading, especially if the books were on an interesting topic. The library was one of my favorite places in the school to go to, whether I was there doing research for a project in one of my classes or just looking for a book that I could read. There was one project we did on the lighthouses of America that I remember finding particularly compelling. We not only learned the facts about the lighthouses, like their name, location, and appearance, but also their significance in American history. Lighthouses symbolize the way forward and help in navigating our way through rough waters. Nothing else speaks of safety and security in the face of adversity and challenge quite the way a lighthouse does. I also liked it when we got to choose what we wanted to read ourselves. It was expected that we would read a certain amount on our own at home, as part of our homework. Every student had a paper to fill out with the number of pages they read each night, along with the name of the book and how long it took us to read it. Reading a few pages became one of my regular pre-bed activities.

Reading was a wonderful way to learn new words, although we worked on vocabulary separately, too. We would be given lists of words every so often and were expected to memorize their meanings. My dad would sometimes quiz me on the new words I was learning to make sure I was making good progress. I made it a point to learn at least one new English word every day, and unlike the Spanish vocabulary which I learned and then later forgot, I still remember most of these words, even the long ones I didn't use very much, like "bewilderment."

Understanding what words mean is important, but just as important is knowing how to spell them correctly, and we worked on that in class, too. Every year the school held a "spelling bee" for its students, to test out which of us was the most knowledgeable in this regard. My 3rd grade year was the first time I'd competed in any kind of spelling contest like this. At home the night before I watched a special movie, called *Akeelah and the Bee*, to inspire me to be my best during the contest the next day. I was eliminated from the spelling bee fairly early, but it was still amusing getting to be a part of the competition.

Along with learning the mechanics of the English language like spelling, vocabulary, and grammar, we also worked on putting them all together into a story. In third grade, my teacher—Ms. Judd—would have us lie down in a designated corner of the classroom while she read us stories. By fourth grade, when I was taught by Ms. Norman, we had story writing time, too, and sometimes even switched classrooms when it was time for our English class. We could write about whatever topics we wanted, and the teacher encouraged us to expand our minds as much as possible and let our imaginations run wild, putting together magical elements with more realistic ones and being creative with all of our choices. She would read our stories and suggest what we could do to make them even better. One correction I remember was to the way I ended my stories. When I first started writing stories, I was in the habit of writing "The End" at the bottom of the last page every single time. I later understood that this was a cliché and I shouldn't do it; a reader would be smart enough to recognize that the last line of the story was the end. Slight changes like that helped all of the students to create better stories.

The more mathematical and scientific classes were also interesting for me and offered a lot of different new experiences. We had computer sessions where we would learn to type using a site called Dance Mat typing. Even after coming back to India I still practice my typing and advise others who want to learn to type to go on the site. In math class, we learned a whole bunch of different terminology related to the field. We would use index cards to learn these terms, which we kept in alphabetical order in a little tin box. Every day we would write out a new card, with a new term or expression for us to learn. Sometimes during the class, we would be taught using a projector, or were called up to the front of the class to solve a sum.

The science classes were a whole new experience for me. We watched videos explaining astrological bodies, like the sun and the moon, including the one that showed the Earth revolving around the sun. We also did a lot of different hands-on experiments that helped us to learn all the concepts and ideas in a more interesting way than just reading about them in our textbooks. An experiment that I remember vividly was a test we did on marshmallows in fourth grade to see if they contain starch. The teacher divided us into groups and put each group at its own table. Each table had a plastic container that could be used to hold pieces of the marshmallows that the teacher passed around. We took a piece of marshmallow, put it in the container, then put a few drops of iodine in it and mashed it together. The iodine was a light brown liquid, but it turned blue-black when it was dripped onto the marshmallow, indicating the marshmallow contained starch. These kinds of experiments were a great way to see how the world worked.

There were so many different things to love about Creekside Elementary. The teachers and staff went out of their way to make sure every student felt accepted and welcomed, no matter where they were from or how long they'd been attending the school. When it was a student's birthday, their name was read during the morning announcements, and their teacher would give them a hug and a special pencil. My eighth birthday fell on a school day and I was able to have a party in the school itself. My dad and Seema came in with packets of chips and boxes of juice for my entire class to enjoy. It definitely made me feel very special, having all of my friends from the school wishing me happy birthday. We had a separate celebration that night at home, too, complete with a cake, which I was supposed to cut all by myself.

I loved going to school in the US. Every day brought new adventures and was full of fun. Despite my shyness and the fact that I didn't talk much, I made a few good friends while I was going to school at Creekside. My friend Daniel was a pretty girl with short hair. I went to her home with her on the bus at least once, and we played basketball together until my dad picked me up. I also had a close friend named Amelia. She was the first person in America to invite me to a birthday party. This was my first experience with an American birthday celebration. In India, birthday parties are often much bigger in scope, with 50 or more friends and relatives in attendance. Even smaller gatherings were usually highly organized, with scheduled snacks and games and a gift exchange at the end. Amelia's birthday party was smaller, just a few friends. Her mother took us to a bowling alley—my first time bowling, also—and we had pizza and drinks while we played. Afterwards we went back to her house and ate an American-style dinner, playing songs and games until our parents came to pick us up.

There were people at the school from all over the world. My school friend Yaqoub was maybe the only kid I met in America who could pronounce my name right. I had a few Spanish friends I'd play with during recess, running around the slides and swings. I remember Madeleine most for how beautifully she could hum. I had another classmate who was from Vietnam. I hadn't heard of this country before I met him, and it was exciting to learn about this new place in the world. Some of my friends lived in the Copper Ridge apartment complex where we lived, like my friends Travis and Connor. The ones that went to Creekside, like my friend Chancellor, rode the same bus as me. One girl, Rachel, taught me how to play Mancala and gave me the game board; I enjoyed playing it with my dad. In the winter time, Abhinav would come to visit and he'd play outside in the snow with me and my friends from the complex.

One of my American friends was a boy named Davis. His mother, Professor Julie Clerque, met my dad during a fundraising event at the school. She heard my father using Hindi terms when he answered a phone call. She smiled broadly and greeted my father in the Indian way, by saying, "Namaste ji."

My dad was pleasantly surprised to hear someone speaking Hindi. "How do you know the Indian greeting?" he asked. It turns out she'd spent a few years in Banaras, India during the 1970s, doing research for her thesis in Public Health. She now worked as a research Fellow and Investigator at the University of North Carolina's Sheps Center for Health Services. I already enjoyed playing with Davis, so it made sense that my father and Julie would become fast friends, too.

From their first meeting on, the relationship between our family and the Clerques was strong. Ms. Julie invited all of us (my dad, Abhinav, Seema and me) to her home for dinner. Abhinav was visiting at the time so he came along, too. The Clerques had a beautiful mansion, but what I was most excited about was Davis's hamster. It was the first time I'd seen one. I couldn't believe how fluffy it was, like a cute, chubby little mouse. While the hamster was the highlight, I also enjoyed playing Wii tennis with Davis and eating the delicious Indian food Ms. Julie served us.

Julie and Davis weren't the only new friends we met during our two years living in North Carolina. The McClellands were another family we became close to during our stay. This was the family of Mr. Rob McClelland, the guardian of my daily bus ride to school. Mr. Rob is a warm and gentle man with a big heart, and his wife, Mrs. Barbara, shares these qualities. By the time I was in fourth grade, both my dad and I felt like the McClellands were part of our own extended family. There would always be big hugs whenever we met. We went over to the McClelland house for dinner sometimes, as well. The first time we went they made a meal of rice and pinto beans, with fresh applesauce that Barbara had made herself for dessert. After eating applesauce at the McClelland house, the dish became a staple for our family, too. My dad still occasionally makes applesauce with green apples. One time I vividly remember him making it was when I got my braces, in 2013, and had trouble eating more solid food. We would sometimes eat out with the McClellands often at the UNC Club. From our family, it would be Seema, my dad, and myself, as well as my brothers if they were around; from theirs, Mr. Rob and Mrs. Barbara, along with their daughter Megan, her husband Andrew, and their children, Asher and Charis.

Along with the friends my dad and I made in North Carolina, my brothers would come to visit a lot while we were there. Abhinav wasn't living in the United States anymore at this point, having moved to London the semester before my dad's appointment began, but he still managed to visit us in Chapel Hill twice while we were there, once in 2008 when we were first setting up our apartment and again in 2009. He stayed longer on his second visit because he was preparing to enter law school, getting his applications put together for schools in the United States while he studied to take his LSAT exams. We'd always shared an interest in experimenting with new, unique cuisines, so any time he was around we would go out to eat at all the diverse kinds of restaurants we could find, from Italian to Thai. Sometimes it was fun to go to the local Indian restaurants and get a taste of home. I always made sure to get the mango lassi when we did, which was one of my favorite sweet treats. Abhinav was quite a good cook, too, and he loved making unique vegetarian dishes for us to eat. Abhishek was still living in Boston—not exactly right next door, but just a few hours away. My dad and I sometimes visited him there, while other times he came to North Carolina. Any time Abhinav came, he made sure to test me on my school work. He was always much stricter about this than my dad was, making sure that I could clearly give him the exact definition of whatever term he was quizzing me on.

One of the main things I remember about my time living in North Carolina is that there was always something to do. In the summer when I was out of school, we'd visit Jordan Lake, a beautiful reservoir close to where we lived where you could do all kinds of different fun outdoors activities and enjoy the sunshine. In the winter, I loved playing in the snow that fell in our complex. I'd build snowmen or make snow angels. One time I made a snow angel by laying on the snow and swinging my arms around back and forth. When either Sonu Bhaiya or Abbu Bhaiya were in town, I loved going to the gym with them and getting on the treadmill. We used to go for a swim or to play a sport like basketball. When Abhinav was around, we would usually play tennis together. Even if I didn't have a chance to play whatever sport they were engaged in, I enjoyed hanging out and watching them.

Maybe my favorite place of all, though, was Chuck-e-Cheese's. If you've never been to one of these establishments, they're basically a combination of a pizza restaurant and an arcade. There were tons of different games to play. If you played them well enough, the game machines would give out tickets that could be redeemed for candy and other prizes. I loved competing in the games against Seema or my brothers, whoever was able to come with me on that particular day. I would save up my tickets from the entire day then use them at the end to pick out a selection of toys. Just as much as the games we played I remember the smell in the air, how it was both fresh and sweet. In my mind, this aroma is still the smell of childhood fun. My dad liked Chuck-e-Cheese's too, I think, because he got to relax while I played with Seema or my brothers. Also, he was quite fond of playing "Deal or No Deal".

My two-year stay in the United States was full of memorable moments. I was certainly sad to go when my father's assignment ended and it was time to pack up all of our things and return to India. It was the spring of 2010 when our time at UNC came to a close. Abhinav had been staying with us still while he waited for the results of his LSAT, which he received in March of 2010, just in time for the end of my dad's appointment as an International Visiting Scholar. Seema was still finishing up with her graduate studies, so she remained behind for a few months to complete her degree. Ms. Barbara McClelland heard we were looking for a place for Seema to stay in the US for a couple of months after our departure. She firmly put her foot down and ordered that Seema live with them till the end of her term. Thus, we left Seema with our car, a Nissan Pathfinder, disposed of all our other house-hold items, and moved to India in March 2010.

My teachers seemed as sad to say goodbye to me as I was to be leaving. When I went in to the school for my last day of fourth grade, my teachers gave me a few different going away presents. One gave me a piece of Micah, a rare precious stone that's formed as a result of many thin layers of closely related material; Ms. Norman gave me chocolate coins and a Bugs Bunny stuffed with candies that I still have. Their hugs were warm and comforting. My friends came to the front door to see me off and say goodbye. Although I did not talk much, the friends who came to see me off at the door had tears in their eyes. This moved me a lot. I'll never forget that moment. I was sad to be leaving but felt so touched and blessed by their attention. I couldn't help missing America when I returned to India. I spent a lot of time wishing those days would come back again, and still think fondly on them whenever I look back. I had no way of knowing at the time that I would be returning to the United States in a few short years, albeit for a much less enjoyable reason. At least Abhinav was able to return to Chandigarh with us, even if he would surely be leaving again soon now that he knew the results of his law exam. Having my family around me made returning home to India a much more enjoyable prospect.

Chapter 5

My dad and I moved back to Chandigarh at the end of March 2010. It was a bit before the culmination of the semesters in the United States, but since my father's program was flexible and the Indian school year started in April, it was a logical time for us to leave. Seema finished her degree, graduating with Cum Laude honors, then joined us in India in May. As much as I was sad to leave my friends in North Carolina, it was also nice to see our beautiful city again and settle back into our old routine. I was about to enter fifth grade by this point, so my father enrolled me once again in the Chandigarh branch of Delhi Public School (DPS). My class teacher, Ms. Neelam, was very nice and welcoming, and so were the other students in my class. Even though I had attended the school before, until part of 3rd grade, I was a bit timid since it was a new class. Having classmates who were kind definitely made the transition easier.

It was an adjustment coming back to DPS after having my two years at Creekside, but just like after we moved to North Carolina, it didn't take too long for me to settle into a routine, although my routine in India was a bit more hectic than the one I'd followed in the United States. My bus would pick me up as early as 7 in the morning and drop me off at home around 2:30 in the afternoon. I'd have lunch before starting my studies. Six days a week I would have an hour of tutoring, alternating between studying math and science. I would be finished with tutoring around 5pm. If I was still feeling energetic I'd go to a nearby park with Seema, but a lot of times I would be completely exhausted and would instead start in on my homework so I could finish it before I went to sleep. Once a week or so my dad and I would go out for dinner at a club or hotel restaurant with an assortment of family friends, something that always reminded me of going to the dinner clubs at UNC.

As a grade school student in the United States, it was a bit unusual that I had a tutor after-school for a class I wasn't required to take, like Spanish. Typically, the only students who would use tutors at this age in the United States fell into one of the two extremes—either they were struggling and needed the extra help to pass their regular classes, or they were in gifted programs that had them working on more advanced material than they would be covering in their regular school day. When I started fifth grade in India, many of my fellow students went to tutoring sessions after school, just like I did, regardless of where they stood in the class rankings.

The way the teachers acted toward the students was different at DPS than it had been at Creekside Elementary. In the United States, teachers were more soft spoken and discrete when they needed to correct a student. They frequently offered a sympathetic ear for any issues the child was having at home, willing to work with both the student and their parents to resolve them. Teachers in India, on the other hand, tended to use harsher tones when reprimanding students If a student acted up it would earn them a trip to the principal's office, where they would be far more seriously reprimanded than by the teacher (and could even face suspension from school) —and which would undoubtedly also mean a call to the parents. That's something that could happen in the United States, too, although with how much more strict everything in the school tended to be, it sounded a lot scarier in Indian schools.

This isn't to say that Indian school teachers are mean to the kids without cause, or that they were particularly more strict than the other authority figures in a student's life. The parents in India tended to be strict, too. This was why one of the most severe threats that the teachers could make when a student misbehaved was to say that they planned to call the student's parents and tell them that the student had been acting up. It wasn't uncommon for kids to fear their parents' punishment, which could be a simple scolding, getting grounded for a time, or other similar kinds of things. This wasn't the case with my dad—he had never been particularly strict with me, maybe because I was a quiet kid who enjoyed school and didn't need much in the way of reprimanding—but my dad was more the exception than the rule.

This was honestly true with my teachers, too. While I could see that the teachers were generally stricter with other students at the school than the ones in the United States had been, I didn't experience this difference quite as much for myself. I was a bit of an unusual student since I had just come back from spending two years in school in the United States. I was also further along in my studies than many of my classmates. Of the 40 or so people in my class, I was consistently in the top five.

The way the teachers interacted with the students wasn't the only difference between American and Indian schools. In the United States, there's a lot of emphasis on participating in extracurricular activities like sports or music, from the grade school all the way up through high school. That isn't as much of a focus in schools in India, where the academic subjects are more of an emphasis. Most of the parents are far more concerned with their children scoring well on their exams than they are with the creative or athletic activities they participate in on the side.

There are five main subjects in the schools in India. Many of them are similar to classes I took in the United States. Math and English were basically the same, and we also had a Hindi class that was similar to the grammar and reading classes in an American classroom. There is one subject in schools in India called Environmental Studies or EVS for short, that combines the social and physical sciences into one course. Topics like history and geography were covered in this course along with other fields of science. The last main subject is a third language. When it was time for me to sign up for my third language before starting fifth grade, I had the choice of German, French, Sanskrit, or Punjabi. This was a bit of a bewildering choice for me because I didn't know anything about any of these languages. Whichever language I chose, I would have to pick it carefully, because I would be stuck with it for a few years. There wouldn't be an option for me to change the language until I made it to the ninth grade. Since I had already taken Spanish lessons in third and fourth grade in the United States, I decided to pick French, which I knew was very similar.

I always really enjoyed eating lunch in the cafeteria at my school in North Carolina. There were always a lot of different meals to choose from, with options for both vegetarians and meat eaters. It was a large enough space where everyone could eat together, with the teachers in the same area as the students—even parents could eat there, if they wanted to. The entire lunchroom process seemed more organized and systematic. The week's menu would be posted online so students knew what their options would be before they went to school. Every student had an account they used to pay for their meals so they wouldn't have to worry about carrying cash with them to school. At DPS, there was a small canteen for buying food. It sold soft drinks, juices, and snacks, along with a meal prepared by the canteen worker. This would change daily but there was no way to find out ahead of time what the day's meal would be. Getting through the food line was also more chaotic. I wasn't a huge fan of the canteen food, anyway, so I more often would just bring my own food from home.

Maybe the biggest difference I noticed between Creekside Elementary School in the United States and DPS Chandigarh was the amount of homework I had to complete each night. Every class gave us homework to complete pretty much every night, along with weekly tests to study for. These tests were usually on Monday mornings, so I would often spend my weekends at home learning and memorizing the material. Many of my classes at Creekside did assign homework, but it was relatively light—maybe a few easy math problems to practice on a worksheet or some vocabulary words to study and memorize. Some classes had the students complete online assignments but even this wasn't too much work. The most time-consuming work we had to do outside of class was usually our reading, which for me was honestly more fun than work most of the time. I always loved going to the library and picking out interesting books to read. I even enjoyed working on the more extensive long-term assignments that we were given, like the one I mentioned in the last chapter about the lighthouses of America, or another one I remember completing on the science behind rainbows. These projects never felt like a burden when they were assigned at my American school, but the same style of project assigned in my Indian school was quite tiring.

We would even get lots of homework assigned over our school breaks, especially the summer holiday. Some of these would be group projects that we could work on with our friends, but more often it was individual work. For English class, for example, we would often have to read a book and then write a summary of it. Even though we didn't have an official PE class in grade school at DPS, we would sometimes have physical fitness homework to do. I quickly learned that if I decided to treat the homework like it was interesting it wouldn't be as boring. I would always try to get something out of it because of this, helping the time spent doing it to go faster. I took the same approach to the homework assigned on summer holidays, completing it as quickly as I could so I could relax the rest of the summer.

While the teachers in India assigned more homework than the teachers I'd had in the United States, they didn't seem quite as concerned with how the students were completing it. There was one assignment I remember that involved creating a poster to promote carpooling, which I had to hang up in a public area then photograph to prove that I had posted it. We were also supposed to speak with a few people, explaining the project to them and getting them to sign a sheet saying they supported the idea. I actually visited a few of my neighbors and talked with some family friends, though when I got to school and saw the other students' sheets, I noticed they just wrote out comments on a sheet of paper themselves and signed each one with a different name. The same thing happened when we were assigned EVS homework to visit an orphanage. My dad and I visited an orphanage established by Mother Teresa so I could write down my experiences there. Talking to my friends, I found out that none of them had actually gone to an orphanage, instead making up the experience from their own imaginations. I always stayed true to myself, though, and did every task sincerely.

I wasn't sure that I would ever make good friends or be able to mix it up with my classmates when I started back at DPS, since I was a bit of an introvert, but the students in my class who befriended me quickly made me feel like I was home again. They taught me how the time table and schedule for the school ran, helping me to figure out what I had to do when. All of the group projects we were assigned in the school made me interact with more of my classmates, helping us to get to know each other and making it easier for me to communicate with them. It took a little while, but gradually I started being more social.

Though we didn't have a formalized PE class at DPS, we did still have a recess time where we were set loose to run around the playground. Sometimes we'd just run around, but other times we'd form up into groups and play games. One of our favorites when I was younger was a game similar to the American game of tag but with the added detail that each kid would choose a name from any category (say animals/fruits/cars, etc.) to refer to themselves as, and the person who was "it" (called the "diner") would announce who was to be tagged next by saying the name of the animal. There were other fun games to play, too. I also joined the morning sports class, which was taught by Tejinder Sir from 6:30am to 7:30am. My best friend and classmate, Damini always attended morning sports with me. We'd warm up by stretching and running, then he'd teach us proper basketball techniques (like chest pass, lay-up, rebound, etc.). I was glad that Damini came with me to the classes, since it was attended by more boys than girls and most of them were older than we were.

I loved learning and going to school just as much at DPS as I had back at Creekside Elementary. The only subject that sometimes gave me trouble was EVS, which I often had to cram for if I wanted to do well on the tests. Even though I enjoyed school more than most kids, I still looked forward to my summer vacation, especially since that meant I would be able to go on trips. Every summer, the school would organize a class trip. The holiday after fifth grade, the 15 or so students in my class went to Goa, a state in western India with coastline on the Arabian Sea that's known for its tropical beaches, spice plantations, and fishing villages. It was my first time going on a trip without anyone from my family and even though there would be teachers there, my dad was concerned about me traveling alone. He sent Abbu Bhaiya along with me in case there was an emergency, though my brother stayed at a different hotel and out of my hair for the most part.

I was a bit nervous about this class trip to Goa, even as we boarded the bus to Delhi, where we would be catching our flight to Goa. Only two of the students were from my section and the rest I didn't know very well, so I wasn't sure if I would have fun and feel comfortable around them. By the time I saw the glittering 5-star hotel we'd be staying in, though, I knew I'd made the right choice in coming. The hotel was next to a beautiful beach, surrounded by tall palm trees. My room was on the hotel's ground floor and had three separate small beds for the three students who'd be sleeping there. The first night we went to a fantastic dinner, then later went out to the deck and danced in our pajamas.

The next day we took a tour of Goa. The streets were very narrow, made more so by the vendor stalls set up along them. There was one vendor who put on temporary tattoos, like stamps, and another who sold coconut water and coconut cream fresh from the fruit, cut right in front of customers' eyes. Me and some of the other students used the pocket money our parents had given us to purchase the things the vendors had on offer. Our second morning in town, we played on the beach at the back of the hotel. I'd worn my favorite fancy black slippers, which turned out to be a mistake. While we were playing tug of war in the sand, my slippers broke, and I realized too late I should have taken them off before playing. Other students lost their shoes to the current in the water, so it was apparently an unlucky day for footwear.

That afternoon we shifted collectively to the swimming pool. I was swimming with my friends when I saw my brother walking toward me. I was a bit confused and unhappy to see him. I knew I hadn't done anything bad on the trip, so I approached with my usual innocent smile, not sure why he was calling me to get out of the pool and come talk to him. It turned out that the teachers had noticed me loaning out my phone to the other kids so they could call their parents at home. I didn't see any problem with doing that; after all, if the situation were reversed, I would want someone to let me borrow their phone so I could talk to my dad. Abbu Bhaiya explained that it cost more to use our phones here than at home because of roaming charges and told me not to lend my phone out too often or else the other kids might take advantage of my generosity.

The trip to Goa lasted a total of five days and ended up being one of my most memorable trips, especially compared to other school trips I would take. The flight home wasn't my favorite, though. I was used to international flights, where everyone got a meal, but this was a domestic flight, where we didn't get any free food. After the flight to Delhi there was still the bus to Chandigarh. I was exhausted by this point and fell asleep during the ride. When we finally got back to the school and my dad picked me up, I was too tired to even talk to him, and went straight to my bed as soon as we got home.

Later in the summer, my dad and I decided to renew the tradition of visiting my brother in the United States during my vacation. Just like we'd done in previous years, we visited family friends, went to theme parks, and had a lot of fun sight-seeing. I especially loved going shopping—there was so much variety in the stores. This trip was even better than the ones I'd taken in past years since I was old enough to enjoy and remember more of the things that we did. I also decided not to attend the summer camps in the United States I'd gone to in the past, instead spending that time working on my summer homework and hanging out with my family.

By the time I went back to school for sixth grade I was feeling much more comfortable with my teachers, classmates, and school than I had at the start of the previous year. Ms. Geeta, who had a background in computers, was our class teacher. My home tutor for sixth grade was Ms. Anjana, who would come to my home and help me study everything I had learned in all my school subjects that day. One of my neighbors who also studied in the same grade at DPS, a friend named Sakshi, attended the tutoring sessions with me. After tutoring, sometimes we would go to the park and walk, or play badminton together with Seema or another neighbor, Nannie, who was just a year ahead of us at a different school. Other times I would go to Sakshi's house so we could play or study together.

My sixth-grade year flew by and soon enough it was time for the summer holiday and our next organized school trip. This time my class was going to Agra, the home of the Taj Mahal—one of the seven wonders of the world. We went straight to the hotel the first night then the next morning went to see the Agra Fort and Fatehpur Sikri Fort. It was a grand building, with the rooms open on both sides, which the guide of our tour explained to us was the way the builders kept the rooms cool in the time when there were no fans and air conditioners. They would also put a large bowl of water and rose petals under the bed to help cool the room and give it a nice, floral aroma. The fort was absolutely magnificent, with elaborate designs carved into the ceilings, but it still paled in comparison to our next stop: the Taj Mahal. That palace was so grand that it took 22 years to build it, constructed by the Mughal Emperor Shah Jahan as a memorial to his late wife, Mumtaz Mahal; a wide passage connected Mumtaz' tomb to the main room of the Taj Mahal. The palace was constructed of white marble, both inside and out. It must have been an absolute marvel to behold when it was first built, though by the time we visited it had lost a lot of its beauty due to the air pollution of the city. The hotel we stayed at in Agra was nice, too, with a great breakfast buffet and souvenir shops on the ground floor. I enjoyed browsing them, though I didn't buy anything—except a nice scarf for Seema—during our four-day trip.

For the next year, Sakshi and I changed to a new tutor. Her name was Ms. Vinita and she lived nearby, only around a five-minute walk from our neighborhood. She tutored us in math and science from the school-prescribed book published by the National Council of Educational Research and Training (or NCERT for short). Ms. Vinita was a bit stricter than my last tutor had been, and she even gave additional homework, but she was a superb teacher who really helped me to develop my knowledge in those subjects.

During my seventh-grade year my class teacher was Ms. Roma. We had a food festival to celebrate the different regional cultures and cuisines of India. The class was divided into eight sections, each of which was assigned a different Indian state to depict. My section was to research and depict the state of Kerala, which is on the south-west coast of India. The other students in my group and I brought food related to the area and materials to decorate the classroom with. Some of the girls in my group wore the region's traditional cream-colored saree, though I chose not to wear this traditional dress, instead bringing banana leaves in for us to serve the food on. At the end of the food festival, we all had a dance party in our classroom.

Ms. Roma is a very enthusiastic teacher. While Ms. Roma was my classroom teacher, we had additional teachers for other subjects. For English class, my teacher in seventh grade was Sangeeta mam. While I liked many of my teachers and found them very kind and nurturing, Sangeeta mam is an especially beautiful soul. We formed such a tight bond during my seventh-grade year in her class that in eighth grade and onward I would sometimes go to her classroom and hang out with her on my lunch breaks. We still keep in contact with each other, talking on the phone every now and then.

My seventh-grade class trip was to Jaipur, Rajasthan, also called the Pink City. In the previous year I had come out of my shell a bit and made quite a few new friends. More students from my section were going on the trip, as well, which made me even more excited for this trip than I had been for the previous two. Having the experience of my previous class trips, I decided to pack all of my things into my backpack, which made it much easier to roam around. This time instead of a bus or plane we were taking a train to get there. I started in a window seat, talking to my friends for a while, then moved back to the sleeper car when I started to get tired. I was supposed to sleep on the top bunk, but I was afraid I would fall out during the night, so my friend who was sleeping in the bed below me said I could sleep with her for the night. Once I felt safe and secure, sleeping on the train was very peaceful. The view out of the window was beautiful and relaxing, and the moon was shining in the night sky. It was a long journey to Jaipur; we changed trains the next day, then finally took a bus to our hotel.

Compared to other hotels I had stayed at, I didn't find the food at our hotel in Jaipur very good. In fact, I decided not to eat lunch that first day, instead waiting to eat until we went to Chokhi Dhani, a resort in Rajasthan with rides, vendors, and shows. For dinner, they served us traditional Rajasthani food like dal (lentil), baati (Rajasthani bread), and churma (crushed bread blended with sugar). There was also a cola stand, where we could get flavored ice made with a variety of different syrups. The shows and lights were superb and we all had a great time. By the time we got back to the hotel, I was dead tired and went straight to sleep. The next day, we took a tour of Amer Fort, a beautiful mountaintop fort about 11 kilometers from Jaipur, near to Maota Lake. We took three-wheeled bikes called rickshaws up the mountain to the palace. While there, we learned all about the history of the fort and looked at the beautiful Hindu architecture. It was built of red sandstone and marble, with multiple courtyards outside. The rooms in the fort were very wide, but the acoustics of the space were such that you could call out to someone from a specific place in the room and the other person could reply from the other side, without raising their voice.

We saw other sights on this trip, as well. After leaving the Amer Fort, we went to a planetarium. We also drove the three hours from Jaipur to Bharatpur where there was a famous bird sanctuary. It was designed like a sprawling forest, with a narrow passage between the trees for the visitors to travel down. Rather than going through the sanctuary as one large class, we split up into smaller groups and each one was given a guide with a pair of binoculars who could help us spot the various birds we encountered as we went. It was impressive how the guides could pick the birds out of the thick foliage and trap them in the binocular's sight so all the kids could get a close-up look at them. By the time we'd finished going through the entire sanctuary it had gotten quite dark, so we hopped onto our bus and made our way back to the hotel. After visiting a few shops, I bought a beautiful hand-made scenery painted on black paper and a small nice marble container. A couple days later we took the train back to Chandigarh. Like when I came back from past trips, my dad was there to greet me at the station and bring me home.

Between my trips to America with my family and the various trips I took with my school, I had already traveled quite a bit and had many remarkable experiences by the summer of 2013. Having made many new friends during the previous school year, I was especially excited to start eighth grade the following school year—even more so than I normally was, and I'd always been much more passionate about school than most kids. I was already thinking about the important exams I had coming up even as I finished my summer homework, excited about what the next year would bring. Little did I know that there was a new challenge on my horizon, one far greater than simply another year of classes that would drastically alter the course of my future over the coming years.

Chapter 6

After the summer of 2013, my attention shifted immediately to my approaching half-yearly exams. The tests themselves would be taking place in late August, but the intense studying for them started a month before. I could feel their approach like a tension hovering in the air around me; I knew how vital good scores would be to the future of my education, which had always been very important to me.

I started feeling unwell about this time. Sometimes anxiety can lead to stomach aches and other physical problems, but I knew this was more than just nerves. On August 5th of 2013 the pain in my stomach became particularly severe and I complained to my father about it. His mind must have turned to my mother's health issues fifteen years before, which had started with similarly severe abdominal pain. He contacted Dr. Sarla Malhotra, who had been one of the doctors overseeing my mother's treatments. She had retired from PGI in the intervening years and was now working as a senior consultant at Fortis Hospital in Mohali. My dad set up an appointment with her and immediately sent me and Seema to her home.

I have always felt an extraordinary bond with Dr. Sarla. In some ways I owe my existence to her. When my mother first realized she was pregnant and when there was still some uncertainty about whether I would have a chance of being born healthy, Dr. Sarla was the only figure in the medical community who firmly believed my mother should give birth, whatever may happen in the end. I could think of no one I trusted more to diagnose the source of my stomach pain. After examining me and hearing me describe my symptoms, Dr. Sarla advised me to get an ultrasound taken. Even she said that normally when young girls complain about stomach pain, it would be usually due to menstruation or digestive problems. She never normally would have requested an ultrasound. With me, she felt that God had told her to recommend me to get the test done.

The evening after I received the ultrasound, my father met with Dr. Sarla to go over the report. They asked me to wait in another room while they discussed it—evident enough what it had revealed was serious, even if I hadn't seen the grim look on Dr. Sarla's face. The radiologist had confirmed there was a tumor in my ovary and suspected it could be malignant. It was Dr. Sarla's advice that I get further tests taken, including tests for cancer markers like Alpha Fetoprotein (AFP) and CA 125.

My dad didn't explain any of these details to me that day at Dr. Sarla's home. The only thing Dr. Sarla said to me after her private conversation with my dad was that I should stay home from school for a couple of weeks. A lot of kids probably would have been excited—any excuse to stay away from school would do. Not me, though. I was shocked. I loved going to school and didn't want to miss my classes, especially with the half-yearly exams approaching. How was I supposed to prepare for my exams if I couldn't go to class and study? It wasn't until later that night my dad explained the situation to me. There was a tumor in my stomach, and I would need to have an operation to remove it. He also made sure to tell me this might just be the first step of a longer process. I still didn't completely understand why this meant I couldn't go to school, but I could tell that he wouldn't change his mind on the matter.

When we found out that I would need to have surgery, there was some uncertainty about where I would have the procedure done. The primary options were PGI or Fortis, because they were both relatively close to us, but we considered other options, too. The son-in-law of Mr. Jugal Verma worked at a hospital in Indianapolis and reached out to one of his colleagues there, Dr. Wafic M. El Masri. Mr. Verma sent him my CT scan and report. Dr. Masri examined the report then called my dad and spoke with him over the phone about the procedures involved in surgery. He also sent an email to give more guidance to the doctors in India, helping to clarify what operating methods to follow. Based on the reports, his best conclusion was that I had either an ovarian germ cell tumor or a sex-cord stromal tumor. He believed the tumor was affecting only a single ovary, which made it very important to avoid intra-operative rupturing. This would preserve the health of my other ovary, uterus, and other organs, and prevent me from losing my fertility. He suggested that chemotherapy would be required after the surgery and thought it best for me to get the treatment in the United States. He even suggested it might be best to have the surgery in the United States, if my pain could be adequately controlled with medication.

We initially considered PGI for my surgery, for two main reasons. First, that Dr. Sarla would be able to operate on me there; and secondly, that the operating theater would be available sooner, allowing us to set the date of the surgery more quickly than we would have been able to get in at another institution. PGI was also cheaper than Fortis and was a lot closer, within easy walking distance of our home. Before we made our ultimate decision, we met with Dr. Sarla and another gynecologist to seek their advice about what course of action to take. One option was to get chemotherapy before the surgery, which would reduce the size of the tumor and make it easier to operate on. The problem was that my AFP was very high (a reading of 52,537) and the tumor itself was very large—large enough they were concerned it would burst soon, spreading the cancer throughout my body. This led the doctors to opt for the second option, which was to have me go through surgery first then consider whether or not I would need chemotherapy treatment. Since the operating theater at Fortis was available the next day and there was staff available to meet our needs, the doctors ultimately chose to have my surgery there, rather than PGI as we'd initially decided.

My dad phoned my brothers to tell them about my diagnosis. Abhishek booked the first available flight to India, finding one that would get him there in time for my surgery. When I talked to him on the phone before his flight, he told me he was coming so that he could give our dad emotional support, not just for me, but I was still glad he would be around. Abhinav couldn't make it in person but we spoke on the phone a lot anyway and I knew his thoughts would be with me.

Dr. Sarla wasn't the only familiar face who would be involved in my treatment. Dr. J. D. Wig had been the head of the Gastroenterology department at PGI when my mother went there for her first round of cancer treatments. It was Dr. Wig who had successfully operated on my mother back in 1999. Dr. Wig was now working as a Senior Consultant at Fortis Hospital. When Dr. Sarla went to him asking if he would oversee my surgery, he immediately agreed and began forming a team to work under him. He arranged for the necessary infrastructure to be made available by all concerned departments, in case he should have need of it, and found the earliest available slot in the operating theater to schedule my surgery. His expertise and dedication gave me and my family confidence that my operation would be successful.

I was admitted to the hospital a few days later, the day before my scheduled surgery. All my vitals were checked when I was admitted, and my blood pressure was checked occasionally throughout my first night in the hospital. A lot of different doctors and nurses stopped by to collect information about my medical history, especially related to menstruation. I had a small cough, so they administered steam. I wouldn't be allowed to eat the next day in preparation for my surgery, so I had a hefty dinner: a variety of lentils and vegetables, roti, rice, curd, and salad. There was so much food I couldn't even finish everything.

Back at my school, the day of my surgery was the day of the first half-yearly exam—28th August—on my toughest subject, Social Science. I couldn't help thinking about my friends back at the school preparing for the test and feel anxious about the fact that I would be missing it. I was far more worried about that than I was about the surgery. When I mentioned it to Dr. Wig, though, he and my dad both told me that wasn't something I should be worried about right now. I could retake the exams once the surgery was over. My health was a far more important thing to take care of. I understood what they were telling me and did my best to forget about the exams.

I was a bit jittery on the day of the surgery, but I wasn't scared. I wasn't particularly happy to have to wear the boring blue hospital gown and cap, but I was far more excited about the surgery than you might expect. I didn't know what was going to happen or what the effects would be, and I was eager to find out. Finally, the time arrived. The operating theater was very cold, especially with the minimal protection of my hospital attire. I was given anesthesia through the IV in my hand. It kicked in within seconds. The next thing I knew, the surgery was over. It had taken about three hours and they had successfully removed the entire tumor.

I was then taken to the Intensive Care Unit (ICU) for a few hours to make sure all was well before I would be taken to my private ward. I had awakened from the anesthesia, but I was still feeling very groggy. My eyes kept trying to close, and I couldn't see anything clearly, though I could hear other patients in the ward around me. I could feel that I had a catheter and that my breathing was being assisted by an oxygen mask. My stomach felt sick, and there was a feeling of a lot of pressure on it, too, although I couldn't see the stitches or the incision since they were covered by a white cotton patch. Most of the time I was in the ICU I slept, waking up every thirty minutes or so to look around groggily, feeling terribly nauseous, and fall right back asleep.

Eventually, I was relocated to a private room. Because the risk of infection was high, I wasn't allowed to have many visitors while I recovered in the hospital. My dad was allowed in to see me, of course, and so were Abhishek and Seema, but everyone else who came to see me had to wait out in the lobby. My dad would go out there to meet everyone and thank them for stopping by. He would come in later and tell me about everyone who came by. I was touched to know so many people cared that much about my health, although it was probably for the best that they couldn't come in and see me. I'm not sure that I would have made very good company either. I still wasn't allowed to eat or drink anything and once the anesthesia wore off fully my stomach was in a lot of pain, especially in those first twenty-four hours after surgery. The medication they gave me through my IV dulled the effects but couldn't make it go away completely. The nurses came by often to check on my blood pressure and pulse, making sure I didn't have a fever or any other signs of infection. Sonu Bhaiya stayed by my bedside through all of it during the day.

The tumor was placed in a large jar with fluid to preserve it. My dad drove Abhishek to PGI, where he dropped off the tumor so they could prepare the pathology reports. I never saw the tumor myself, but they showed me photos of it when they came back afterwards to my room at Fortis. It didn't look like much, though—basically just a big lump floating in liquid.

I remained in the hospital for about a week after my surgery. My family made sure I was never there alone. Seema would sit with me in the ward at night, along with frequent daytime visits, and both my brother and my dad were there with me quite a bit. I still wasn't allowed to eat anything solid for the first few days. Anytime my brother would order his lunch into the ward and eat it around me I would watch him longingly, my mouth watering, wishing that I could have some. He explained that all of the nutrition I needed was being given to me through the IV in my hand. I knew that was true, but I couldn't help wishing for just a taste of some of my favorite foods—some of which I knew I wouldn't be allowed to eat for a while.

I enjoyed a lot being in the hospital although I had to keep wearing the same blue hospital clothes. I missed the colorful clothes I'd worn at home and asked my family if they could wear some when they came to see me since I couldn't. My dad's wardrobe was plain, but both my brother and Seema obliged, coming to see me in bright attire that brought a bit of cheer to the ward room. Abhishek also brought me some things from home to make my stay easier, like the stuffed bunny my fourth-grade teacher had given me. It was a great comfort to sleep with at night, so soft and fluffy, and it really helped me not miss home as much. Abhishek also brought a tablet with him when he came to visit to help me pass the time. There was a game on it called Trap that we both loved to play. We would pass the tablet back and forth, competing against each other to see who could reach the highest level. Other times we'd watch cooking shows together and I used to make list on my tablet of the different food items I would gobble down once I was fully recovered. Even when we weren't doing anything in particular, just having Sonu Bhaiya there to talk kept me from getting too bored or restless.

Dr. Sarla stopped in to check up on me almost every evening. Dr. Wig and Dr. Bhushan also came by for regular visits. Seeing my doctors was always a big relief, especially Dr. Sarla, who had such a comforting manner that it would set me right at ease. My recovery progressed well, and after 3-4 days I was ready to start walking again with my nurse's help. There had been an epidermal stuck to my back to reduce my pain, but this was removed after a few days, making it extremely painful to sit up the first couple of times I tried it—even with the nurse's help. Everything was so much harder than I remembered it being. Turning my body so my legs were hanging over the side was difficult, and once I was standing up, it felt like I had crazy legs. I had to take my steps slowly and still kept losing my balance. I felt so clumsy and had to hold on to the nurse's hand to keep from falling, but step by step I made my way around the room. I showed my brother when he came in, excited by my progress—one step closer to going back home.

Even more exciting was when the doctors told me I could start introducing food into my system again. At first, I was only allowed to drink liquids: lemon water, coconut water, and buttermilk were all I was given. Later, I tried eating fruit, but that was a bad idea; it came right back up, along with everything else in my stomach. The doctors waited a couple more days, then had me try taking in some lentils and yogurt. I would also drink plain soup a few times a day. This time I was able to keep it in my stomach. My diet still needed to be carefully monitored, even after I was released from the hospital, but at least I could now eat some of the things I'd been missing.

I could walk again and eat again, and my incisions were healing well. I was allowed to return home to continue my recovery, although I was warned by my doctors not to over-exert myself or try to move around too much, or else I would risk pulling out my stitches. This was hard advice to follow—I was so excited to move around the house that at first I couldn't help myself. The day after I got home, though, I noticed some liquid coming out of the white cotton gauze across the stitches on my belly. My dad took me to the hospital to have it checked out straight away. It was only a bit of pus, a normal part of the healing process, but it made me realize I needed to be more careful to not go up and down the house too much.

Even though I could walk a few steps on my own now, sitting up and laying down were still very difficult tasks, since they meant using the muscles right around the surgery site. Sonu Bhaiya was always there to help me. He would hold me with both hands—one on my back, one supporting the back of my head—then either lift me up or lay me down with utmost care and gentleness. I knew I would be safe whenever bhaiya had me in his arms. Every day I got a little bit stronger. Dr. Sarla called me back to Fortis Hospital a few days after I was released so that she could take out the external stitches; the internal ones would dissolve on their own over time. A couple days after that, I could move around enough to take a full bath without any help. The only big thing I still couldn't do was eat what I wanted to. I still had to just watch Abhishek eat all kinds of delicacies, mouth-watering, living vicariously through his enjoyment of them. The day before his return flight to the United States, Abhishek asked me to order a good pizza for him. When it arrived, the pizza looked and smelled so delicious that I wanted to eat a slice more than anything, but I controlled my temptation. I would have to be satisfied with knowing he had really enjoyed eating it.

Abhishek was able to stay for more than a week after my surgery, but eventually he had to go back. Without my brother, I was just sitting around by myself at home all day, doing nothing. It didn't take long for the boredom to become excruciating. I asked my dad when I would be allowed to go back to school, but he couldn't tell me for sure. We were still waiting to receive the pathology reports from the tumor the doctors had removed from my body during the operation. If I needed more treatment, it could be quite a while before I was able to pick up my old routine.

When the reports did come in, the news wasn't good. They confirmed that the tumor had in fact been malignant, comprised of cancerous cells that could still be living and multiplying in my body. My dad immediately began looking for the best treatment options. In the United States, Abhishek took my pathology reports and tumor blocks to hospitals for consultation. He spoke with the doctors at some of the most highly-regarded medical institutions in his region, including Georgetown University Hospital, John Hopkins University, and Hershey Medical Center, to see what courses of treatment they would follow if I were taken there. My family was determined from the outset that I would receive the best possible care.

The tumor removed from me was a type known as a yolk sac germ cell tumor. It is a very rare kind of tumor, especially in children. They're found in and around the reproductive organs, usually in the ovaries, the testes, or the region at the bottom of the spine, known as the sacrococcygeal area. Because of how and where they usually grow, germ cell tumors are often quite difficult to detect. It's easiest to find them when they grow in the testes, where there will usually be a firm, painless swelling that's visible from the outside. There may be some swelling if the tumor is growing in the sacrococcygeal area, usually at the base of the spine, but this can also often be mistaken for a bruise or infection. The most difficult ones to detect are germ cell tumors growing in the ovaries, where they can get quite large before they're noticed. The most common germ cell tumors in children are sacrococcygeal teratomas, which in the right conditions can even be diagnosed in utero.

Doctors have devised a few different methods for detecting germ cell tumors in the trickier areas of the body. The cells that make up these tumors tend to secrete specific hormones, including alpha-fetoprotein (AFP) and human chorionic gonadotropin (HCG). A blood test looking specifically for traces of these hormones can be one effective way to identify the presence of a tumor. They can also be located using tests like ultrasound, CT scans, or MRIs of the pelvis. Once the tumor has been located, it can be biopsied and examined to determine whether it's cancerous.

The tumor growing in my body had been in my left ovary. It had thankfully been detected on time. My left ovary and left fallopian tube were also removed along with the tumor. This gave me a higher chance for a full recovery. While germ cell tumors do tend to be harder to find, one advantage of a tumor located on the ovary is that they're easier to remove once they have been detected. Removing the entire ovary lowers the chances of the cancer spreading to other regions of the body.

The post-surgery treatment for a germ cell tumor can vary greatly, not just based on the location of the tumor but also the stage at which it was discovered and removed. It was actually a bit unusual that the doctors had surgically removed the tumor before starting any other kinds of treatments. That is often the approach taken when the tumor is in testes, but for those in the ovaries or sacrococcygeal region it's more common to administer chemotherapy first to shrink the tumor, making it easier and safer to remove. Radiation therapy is less common as a treatment but it also may be used, either at the hospital or as an outpatient procedure.

Now that we had received the results of my biopsy, Dr. Sarla took my father and me to the PGI Oncology department to discuss further treatment options. The hallway leading to the doctor's office was narrow and lined with patients. Some were in stretchers, some were in wheelchairs, and some were just sitting on the floor, with nowhere else to go. Seeing patients waiting in a line like that right up to the door of the doctor's office instantly turned me off to receiving treatment at PGI. Since Dr. Sarla had taken us, my dad and I still met and talked with the doctors there, but by the time we left I had decided I would rather get my chemotherapy anywhere the infrastructure and hygiene were better.

We were fairly certain that I would need to receive chemotherapy, though—we just didn't know yet exactly where I was going to have it. The doctors we spoke to in Chandigarh suggested chemotherapy should be started around six weeks following the surgery. This would give my immune system time to recover so I would be strong enough to tolerate the chemo drugs but would still be acting quickly enough to prevent the cancer from spreading further and leading to additional problems. This gave us a solid timeline for how long we had to figure out the right place for my treatment. It was early September at this point, about two weeks out from my surgery—we still had some time to make our decision, but we would have to move somewhat quickly.

While we were researching potential hospitals, Mr. Jugal Verma told us about a place called St. Jude Children's Research Hospital. He had donated to the hospital in the past and thought they might prove a valuable resource for us. St. Jude's is a special hospital located in Memphis, Tennessee that provides cost-free treatment for children with life-threatening diseases. It was named after St. Jude Thaddeus, a figure canonized in the Catholic faith as the patron saint of hopeless causes. The founder, comedian Danny Thomas, established the hospital in 1962 as a fulfilment of a promise he'd made to St. Jude years earlier. The story goes that he'd been struggling to make a living and had a child on the way. He'd prayed to St. Jude to help him find a way to support his family after putting his last seven dollars into a church collection plate. If St. Jude would point the way, Danny promised, he would build a shrine in the saint's name. Danny found a good-paying gig the very next week, and when other successes followed he made good on his promise, establishing the hospital that carries the saint's name.

St. Jude's treats children from around the world. They arrange for the patient and their family to travel to the hospital and stay there during treatment, and the care they provide is always free. The hospital's emphasis on research and finding new methods has allowed them to make remarkable strides in the treatment of childhood diseases, especially acute lymphoblastic leukemia, which is the most common form of childhood cancer. In the fifty-plus years since the hospital was founded, the survival rate for this disease has increased from 4% to 94%. Their impressive contributions to the advancement of childhood cancer treatment immediately caught our eye.

In addition to free treatment for accepted patients, the hospital will also provide free consultations for any disease they have already treated. After learning this, we told Dr. Sarla about St. Jude and she in turn sent them a detailed email, including the complete account of my surgery and full pathology reports. They considered my information at their weekly Solid Tumor Conference and quickly replied with their assessment. Their reply stated that since there was already an established protocol for the type of cancer I had, they wouldn't take up treatment for the case. They did offer their guidance through email and sent a chart that could be used in future treatments. In the opinion of the St. Jude doctors, there was a 50% chance that my tumor would return if I were not given chemotherapy treatments. They suggested two possible avenues for treatment: to wait for the full results of the blood tests to indicate whether there were still any cancer markers in my system (specifically AFP, in my case), or to begin chemotherapy treatments using a combination of drugs known as BEP that's commonly used to treat germ cell tumors in children.

The chart we received from St. Jude's wasn't a guarantee of the type of treatment I would receive, but it was the first time someone had given us an idea of what to expect in the weeks ahead. With this new knowledge in hand we narrowed down our options, reaffirmed in our decision to seek treatment in the United States.

My father reached out to Dr. Nitya Nand, who worked as a Senior Professor at the Post Graduate Institute of Medical Sciences (PGI) in Rohtak. Dr. Nand was an old friend of the family's who had always treated me as if I were his own daughter. He suggested that we set up a consultation with Dr. Shripad D. Banavali, who was the Head of the Department of Medical & Pediatric Oncology at Tata Memorial Hospital in Mumbai. He was the region's leading authority on pediatric cancers and had previously treated ovarian germ cell tumors. He also worked at St. Jude Children's Hospital which is considered as the "Mecca" of Pediatric Oncology. This background and experience made him seem as though he would be the perfect fit for my treatment.

Thus, we decided to travel to Bombay and speak with Dr. Banavali. Another family friend, Mr. L.D. Narwal, spoke with his contacts in Bombay and set up a meeting with the doctor. We immediately arranged a flight to Mumbai. It was myself, my father, Seema, and Mr. Narwal, who had arranged for us to stay at the Police Officers' Mess in Worli, Mumbai so we wouldn't have to rush to find lodgings during our visit. The Officers' Mess is built right on the sea, so that the windows of our apartment overlooked the ocean. We took an evening walk along the beach, which was practically in the building's backyard. The sunrise the next morning was exquisite. I watched it and felt hopeful for what the day ahead of me would hold.

We rode to Tata Hospital in a police vehicle. We went through the preliminary formalities and paperwork then were escorted into the room where we met Dr. Banavali. He examined my reports, discussing them briefly with my father, then asked to see the pathology blocks that had been prepared by PGI. He seemed surprised when we told him we didn't have them with us.

"Aditi's older brother lives in America," my dad told Dr. Banavali as way of explanation. "He has taken the blocks with him to the United States for consultation with doctors there."

"Well if you've already arranged for Aditi to receive treatment in America you should give that first priority," Dr. Banavali replied. He suggested we book the next available flight to the United States. Hearing this, we tentatively decided that my treatment should happen in America, but we still had no idea which hospital had the best doctors and infrastructure for my unique diagnosis.

Another friend of my dad's, who lived in Mumbai, Dr. Lakhan Sinha, reached out and suggested we get a second opinion while we were there. He arranged a meeting with Dr. Sandeep Goyal from the Kokila Ben Ambani Hospital, and we went there to see him the next day. Dr. Goyal was a younger man who'd received his medical training in London. He was smart, kind, and supportive, traits you would look for in any doctor. He spoke with us at length about the treatment options that would be available at Ambani Hospital. The facilities were world-class, and the doctors were exceptional, the majority of them having received training in either the United States or Europe.

Dr. Goyal spoke with a colleague to confirm that they would be able to admit me and discuss the timetable for treatment. We were even able to consult with the doctor who'd be administering the chemotherapy drugs. He was the first of the medical professionals we'd spoken with so far who took the time to educate me on the different methods used to deliver the drugs. Intravenous administration is the most common method, since it lets the drugs be absorbed quickly into the blood stream and carried through the entire body. The dosing, length of treatment, and style of administration could vary greatly, however. For temporary treatments (lasting no more than a few days) an angiocatheter could be used. This would be inserted into a vein on the arm or hand, similar to the IVs for medication and fluids I'd been on after my surgery. For longer treatments, though, there are a variety of other options. The least invasive is a PICC line, which is a plastic catheter that can be placed non-surgically and used for multiple, short chemotherapy sessions over the span of a few weeks or months. More serious and intensive treatments required the use of catheters or port-a-caths that are surgically implanted into the patient's body and can last for years.

This was a sobering thought. The doctors and my dad had explained to me that cancer treatments could be hard, and that I would feel sick for a while before I got better. I hoped that my treatment would be one of the shorter, simpler treatment regimens. I knew my health was important, but I couldn't go back to my friends and classes and old life until this was over.

The doctors were experienced, the facilities were modern and clean—on first inspection, Ambani Hospital seemed like it would be a perfect fit. Unfortunately, after reviewing my files, the doctors said it was too late to admit me. They said I should have started my chemotherapy treatments immediately following the surgery, contradicting the advice we'd received from the doctors at PGI, who'd told us to wait six weeks. We returned to Chandigarh richer in knowledge but still no closer to deciding on a location for my treatment.

Back in Chandigarh, my dad set up another appointment with Dr. Sarla and Dr. Wig. He told them what we'd observed and heard at the hospitals in Mumbai. One thing that still concerned us was that none of the hospitals we consulted with yet in India had given us a treatment plan, or in any way explained what they would be doing if I was admitted. We were as dubious of the operations at Tata Hospital as we had been of those at PGI, and for similar reasons. There had been a huge rush of patients in the hospital when my dad, Seema, and I went for our consultation, a hundred or more patients waiting outside consultant rooms, often squatting on the floor because they didn't even have enough chairs. This didn't inspire confidence in any of us that my treatment would be made a priority, as the risk of infection in that kind of environment seemed high. We didn't notice those issues on our visit to Ambani Hospital, but though it was clean and orderly, it too had its issues. Where the doctors were exceptional, the nurses and support staff weren't often as well-trained.

Beyond these issues, my dad and I had a broader concern with all the Indian hospitals we'd visited. None of them seemed to like sharing information with their patients. The doctor who'd educated me at Ambani Hospital had been a rare exception, and even there we had not been given a full treatment plan or told any details of what specifically would be done for me if I were admitted. There is a sense throughout the Indian health care system that patients and their families do not deserve to know any details of the disease or its treatment. It is privileged information only the experts can be trusted with; the doctor/patient relationship is like that between a boss and an employee, or a father and a child. The doctor gives the rules and the patient is expected to follow them blindly, no questions asked.

None of us were comfortable with this approach. I wanted to know what was happening in my body and what the doctors were doing to treat it. We knew that doctors in the United States took a more inclusive approach to treatment. Information about the illness and the medicines used to treat it is made widely available, and that information is up to date and based on the latest research, ensuring that patients understood all their options, along with the potential benefits and side effects of each treatment. There's more of a focus on the patient's comfort. Pain management is given high priority. Tests are administered promptly when they're needed; when the reports come in, they're given directly to the doctor or nurse, who gives a hard copy to the patient and explains the results and what they mean. I really appreciated this emphasis on educating the patients about their treatment. I knew I would be able to get through the treatment much more easily if I understood what was going on and felt like I was a part of the process.

After discussing all our options, we made our decision. The rush of patients and low supervision of junior staff in Indian hospitals would mean a higher chance of infection. Even Dr. Sarla agreed the facilities in the United States were generally better, even though they administered the same chemotherapy regime. This, along with the different attitude toward treatment, made the United States the better choice. We shifted our focus to finding an American hospital.

Chapter 7

The chart from St. Jude's reaffirmed our decision that I would need to receive chemotherapy. We were pretty sure we would be traveling to the United States to get the treatment, but we were running out of time to make our final decision. While the majority of the doctors we spoke with agreed that it was best for me to wait six weeks after my surgery for my immune system to recover, others thought I should have started it already, and everyone agreed I couldn't afford to put off starting it for too long. The longer I waited, the higher the chance that the cancerous cells would spread and lead to further complications.

On September 26th, 2013 I turned thirteen—officially a teenager. I still wasn't able to go back to class, but the day before my birthday I arranged to meet my friends outside of the school. I had an ultrasound taken earlier in the day, then right after it went straight to DPS Chandigarh to see all of my school friends. It was fantastic to see them after having been away for so long. Many of them had birthday gifts to give me, but it honestly felt like a better present just getting to see and talk to them. It was a bit bittersweet seeing them, too. I missed going to class and being around my friends. I couldn't help but look forward to the day I was well enough to go back.

We'd at least decided that the hospitals in America were overall a better option than the ones in India, so I knew I would be going to the United States—and probably for a long time. Seeing my friends outside the school only seemed to make me miss them more. It was like I was homesick before I even left home. Before we booked our flight to America, I called my friends to see if they'd be able to meet up one more time. They told me there was an Olympiad exam happening at the school that day so I went straight there to pay them a visit. They wished me good luck with my trip to America and my treatments. I felt a lot better afterwards. I was ready now to face the difficult months ahead of me. It was funny—I had been so sad to leave the United States and come back to India after the two years my dad and I spent living in North Carolina, but now that

I was about to go back to the United States, I felt the same way. India had come to feel like home to me again and I couldn't wait until I could come back.

The next week, my dad and I flew to the United States. Sonu Bhaiya met us at the airport in Washington, DC. The very first thing I did when I saw my brother was run up and give him a huge hug. The last time he'd seen me, I was barely able to walk around on my own, but by now I'd built up my strength and was able to do pretty much everything I could before. My diet wasn't regulated as closely anymore, either, so when we got back to his house, he made me an array of different delicacies—a nice flip of all the times I'd had to watch him eat delicious foods when I was in the hospital. We spent our first day in DC, walking around and enjoying the fresh air. I'd visited the city a lot of times before but bhaiya still gave me a little tour, always looking for opportunities to help me expand my knowledge. It was a fun diversion, but I knew it was only a temporary reprieve from the serious affairs to follow.

We had an appointment at Georgetown Hospital the day after our trip to see the city. Abhishek had already given them my blocks and records to examine when he first returned to the United States, but they still took some blood samples and measured my vitals to get a more complete picture of my health. We had a lot of friends in the United States, and many of them had reached out to their contacts in the medical community when they heard about my condition. Dr. Julie (Davis' mother, one of the people we'd met while I was in school at Creekside Elementary) contacted the medical center at University of North Carolina and arranged for us to communicate back and forth with them. Another friend from my Creekside days, Mr. Rob McClelland, sent my pathology reports to Duke Medical Center. One of the people who had reached out to hospitals on our behalf was Seema Verna, who at the time worked as a private consultant and is now the Director of Health Administration with the Federal Government. We knew Seema through her parents, Mr. Jugal and Mrs. Dinesh Verna, who were close friends of my father's. Jugal Uncle was the one who had initially brought St. Jude's to our attention before my surgery. We called her Dinesh aunty because she had always treated me and my brothers like her own family. The Verma family could definitely relate to our situation. Dinesh aunty had recently undergone cancer treatments; she was in remission and recovering.

We were bewildered to find that all of these hospitals had the same problem. None of them would give us even an estimate of what the treatment would cost. Any time we asked, they told us it was an open-ended process. The full cost of the treatment wouldn't be made known to us until after it had ended, and we would have to make periodic payments on our account during the course of the treatment, as well. Most of the people who receive treatment in the United States have health insurance that would cover most of the costs, and often have a pre-established maximum out of pocket limit, so they don't have to worry about the specifics of the billing. For a family like ours, that was visiting from abroad and had limited resources, knowing how much the procedure would cost up-front was necessary. If the payments exceeded our financial resources, it would turn an already rough situation into a nightmare. We couldn't start anything until we knew what to expect.

Just when it seemed we were stuck, running out of time and options, we found a ray of hope. One of our family friends, Dr. Ram Goel, had spoken with several doctors in central Pennsylvania. He consulted with the doctors at the Penn State Health Milton S. Hershey Medical Center and in the pediatric oncology department at Penn State Children's Hospital in Hershey, PA, but it had the same policy regarding giving cost estimates. He then spoke with Dr. Gregory S. Willis, who worked at the Ortenzio Cancer Center at Pinnacle Health in Mechanicsburg, PA—a smaller town that was about an hour's drive from Hershey and just a 30-minute drive from Harrisburg. Dr. Willis was the first doctor who agreed to give us a maximum limit for the expense of the treatment. He wouldn't cut back on the quality of the treatment provided to do so, either. He agreed to follow the treatment plan outlined by the institution of our choosing, whether that was the chart and consultation from St. Jude's, or the plan outlined by the doctors at Hershey Medical Center. After the long hours of searching, we had found the right doctor. We packed up our things and headed to Harrisburg.

We were lucky to have a huge support network that stretched across oceans and national borders. Dr. Ram Goel lived in Harrisburg, where he was a professor at Penn State University. Mr. B.K. Singla flew in from India the following week to give my father and me whatever support we might need. Another family friend, Mr. Ved Goyal, also offered support and any help that we required. Both of my brothers were there too, of course. Whatever challenges we were about to face, I knew I was going to be given the best possible treatment and have the full support of our entire community. Dr. Ram Goel even gave his social security number to guarantee that we would meet the costs of treatment, which we had to do before we could begin. This gave us the confidence to stop thinking so much about the costs and budget and instead just focus on what we had to do to make me well again.

The pediatric oncology department at Penn State Children's Hospital in Hershey was the best in the country after St. Jude's. Combined with its proximity, it was a natural choice. We also learned that there was a program sponsored by the Federal Government involving five different medical institutions around the country, including St. Jude's and Hershey Medical Center. All five institutions were actively exchanging their research, guaranteeing that I would benefit from the latest findings as I began my treatment.

Dr. Ram Goel contacted Dr. Mary Fecile at Hershey Medical Center and arranged for us to have an appointment. It was just a quick 30-minute drive from where we were staying in Camp Hill, PA. My aunt,

Sarla Goel, had a home there, but she was away on a trip to Mumbai, India visiting her kids. Since it was so conveniently located to the medical centers, Sarla Aunty offered to let us use the entire house for our stay.

When we arrived at Hershey Medical Center, the nurse took my vitals in the reception area. We were soon ushered into the doctor's office. At this point in time, there was still some disagreement in the medical community about whether a patient of my age and history should be given chemotherapy at all. Dr. Fecile explained this to me and said that she would start by monitoring my AFP levels before reaching a final decision. If my AFP levels stayed normal, they would not administer chemotherapy.

I felt instantly at ease with Dr. Fecile. She projected confidence and authority in such a way that I felt my health was in very good hands. She also had a young Indian intern in her team of doctors named Dr. Shivani Shah. After talking with her, I learned that her parents lived in Mumbai, in the very same building where Dr. Ram Goel's son, Rohit Goel, was living. It was surprising but comforting to be around someone who knew the same people and places I remembered from back home. We instantly developed a personal rapport with the young intern.

Once again, there was nothing I could do but wait. Dr. Fecile wanted to keep an eye on my AFP levels for at least two weeks before deciding whether chemotherapy would be necessary. There was a slight scare a few days after our consultation with Dr. Fecile when I started to feel a sharp pain in my stomach. I went to the hospital for an ultrasound, but it turned out I was only constipated. My diet was once again restricted to liquids and soft foods, like lentils and yogurt, and the problem was solved. The first time the doctors checked my AFP levels they had decreased. I was happy and hopeful to hear it. If the trend continued, it meant I wouldn't need to receive chemo after all. The next time I went in, though, the news wasn't as good. This test showed a sudden increase in AFP levels. It was such a sharp rise that the doctor suspected the readings may have been faulty and ordered the test be administered again. The second test showed the same results as the first, however. My AFP levels were rising. I would need to receive chemotherapy after all.

Once it was official that I would need treatment, Aunt Sarla cut her trip to India short and returned to the United States to help take care of me. Aunt Sarla is an incredibly loving and caring person. She suffers from several age-related ailments but never lets this stop her from taking care of others. I will have an undying gratitude toward her.

It was very gracious of Aunt Sarla to invite us into her home. The only problem was I didn't like the aura in the room where I was staying. I missed my room back in India. My brother took me to Target and we went on a little shopping spree for things that would make my new bedroom feel more like home. We bought tons of princess, music, and dance posters to decorate the walls, along with an air freshener to keep the air smelling nice. Since my immune system would be compromised while I was receiving chemo treatments, we also bought some hand sanitizers and boxes of Clorox wipes. Everyone who came in could use them to fend off what the doctors called "preventable infections," illnesses caused by common germs that my body would be too weak to fight off.

One thing I did love about the house was that it had a basketball court outside. This made me feel a bit nostalgic for my days playing back at school. I could still remember going to the morning classes with Damini or playing with my friends during games period. My brother bought a basketball and air pump so I could shoot baskets whenever I was bored. It became one of my favorite hobbies during my stay. I practiced things I'd learned in school, like rebounds and lay-ups. I figured even if I didn't have the energy to shoot the ball during my treatments, I could at least dribble the ball and amuse myself passing it between my legs.

The first day of my chemotherapy treatments arrived. It would start early in the day, which meant waking up at 5AM—not an easy task for me, and I was proud of myself that I managed it. The doctors advised me to dress warmly and drink lots of liquids before coming in. This would better prepare my veins for the medicine that would be injected into them.

Pulling up to the hospital, I was shocked by how big it was. Luckily for us there was a parking area close to the Children's Oncology department so we didn't have to walk far to get to where we were going. Entering the hospital was another surprise. The air had a delightful floral aroma, like a garden of roses, not at all like the hospital odor I was familiar with from India. There was even a children's play zone near the reception area with toys and coloring books. The staff was all dressed in funny, colorful clothes that helped cheer up the young patients in the ward. The nurses were so friendly and cheerful that I got to know them quickly. Miss Holly was a jolly young woman who always greeted me with a smile, and Miss Joey was wonderful, too, with a unique haircut that made her stand out from the others. She was kind and helpful and would later train me and my dad how to administer the Neupogen shots I would need between the rounds of chemo administered at the hospital.

Every chemo session started with the nurses checking my vitals, like my weight, temperature, and blood pressure. On my first visit, they also asked me about my medical history—if I was allergic to any drugs, or had anything in my history that would affect the treatment. When it came time for them to insert the IV, they had a hard time finding my veins. The nurse gave me a soft ball to hold and told me to press and release it. To be honest, I was pretty scared about having the IV inserted. I remembered having it done in India, and every time it had hurt a lot. The doctors at Hershey were a lot calmer as they inserted the IV, and swiped it with something that helped me not notice the pain at all. In fact, it didn't hurt a bit, to my surprise and relief.

For the next step I was taken to a large room that contained a huge machine. Since this was the first day of my treatment, I was going to get three different medicines: Bleomycin, Etoposide, and Cisplatin, a combination commonly referred to by the abbreviation BEP. I don't remember the exact order in which they were administered, although I think two medications were given side by side, along with a medication to prevent nausea. That particular drug made me very drowsy, but also jittery at the same time, like there was something popping out of the skin on my arms, legs, and stomach. It got so uncomfortable that it would make me wriggle until my brother convinced me it would feel better if I tried to sleep.

When I woke up, I felt terrible. It was like a war had been going on inside my body while I slept. My dad brought me some crackers to eat, and Sarla aunty brought a pair of furry blue slippers that were perfect for walking around in the winter. They were just what I wanted, and I didn't even have to ask. No matter how bad it felt, I knew my family would be there around me to get me through it.

It was important that I stayed hydrated. The doctors suggested drinking lots of Gatorade and water; there were coolers stocked with various Gatorade flavors in the area with the chemo stations. Of course, drinking so many fluids meant I had to go to the bathroom a lot—and that meant I had to drink more fluids. I never seemed to be hydrated enough when the nurses checked on me. Drinking as many fluids as they wanted me to and eating only semi-liquid foods were difficult tasks for me. It was a long day and time passed painfully slow, but finally I was able to return home, even if it was with the IV still in my arm. The Staff Nurse, Ms. Carol, came by to check up on me. Between her patience and her passion for her job, she was the best nurse I could have asked for.

I was feeling both low and energized when I left the hospital. I was happy to be returning home to my room, with its dance posters and fairy stickers, but the chemotherapy had left me exhausted. A few hours after I got home, I started to have a severe pain in the arm with the IV. I was rushed to the emergency room. The doctors there discovered my vein had been exhausted from having so much medicine pumped into it in one day. It was about ready to burst. The doctors quickly removed the IV and put a warm pack on my arm to help it heal. Boy did that ever feel good!

After this scare, my treatment plan was adjusted. The doctors would remove my IV after the first day, since that was when the most fluids would be administered. The IV would then be re-inserted into my arm and kept there for the entirety of the second and third days. After the third day, a small catheter was put into my left arm so my dad could administer my Neupogen injections. My dad is an efficient person and when it came time for him to administer my first injection, he was a bit quick and harsh about it. Gradually, though, he adjusted his technique to be gentler. The covering they put over my catheter was purple—my favorite color. It protected the catheter well enough from things in the environment, but it wasn't waterproof. This made it pretty tricky for me to clean myself since I didn't dare get water on the dressing.

I decided that I wanted to learn how to do the injections myself for my next treatment cycle. The nurse had my dad come to the lesson with me. He ended up falling asleep; with everything that had been going on since we arrived in the United States, he must have been completely exhausted. He woke up when it came time for him to try it on a dummy. I did it on the dummy, too, then later that day gave the injection to myself in the stomach. It made me nervous doing it at first, but every step had been explained to me in detail, with diagrams that made it clear what I was supposed to do. I realized that it was exactly the same process diabetics used to inject insulin—something that regular people did for themselves on an everyday basis. Once I had done it a couple times and felt more comfortable, I was able to overcome my fear. Starting from the second cycle and every day onward, I was able to do the injections myself at home, even if my dad was always sitting beside me to offer emotional support. The best part of the whole process was at the end, when I would put a Tweety Band-Aid over the injection site. These Tweety stickers and the purple wrapping might be small things, but they certainly made me happy. It was good to have that reminder, that from time to time it was okay for me to be a happy soul even during the chemotherapy treatment.

Over time, I got used to living with the chemo treatments. I was eventually able to bathe myself fully and giving myself the injections was no longer a problem. Most of my problems came from the side-effects of the drugs themselves, especially the nausea and the restlessness. No matter how much I slept, I seemed to feel tired all the time. I still couldn't eat solid foods without vomiting so most of my nutrition came in the form of juices. My dad prepared most of these juices from scratch and didn't let anyone bring in pre-packaged juices. My brother would help him make them sometimes. He always tried to make the flavors interesting, making me a variety of juices including fruits like watermelon, orange, and pomegranate, and vegetables like celery, carrot, tomato, cucumber, and beets. The celery juice tasted especially terrible, and I didn't like the idea of having beetroot, but what choice did I have? I missed eating more interesting foods than just juice, but every time I complained about it, my dad would tell me, "It's your health that's at stake. If you want to keep yourself healthy and fight this monster away, you have to keep having these healthy dishes. They may not be tasty, but they'll keep you safer from the evil germs."

His words were very convincing. I tried to take them to heart. I knew these foods were good for me—but that didn't make them taste any better. I just swallowed everything and tried not to let it touch my tongue, something that proved to be more difficult than I would've thought.

My second chemotherapy cycle started on November 7th, 2013. It was Sonu Bhaiya's birthday. We celebrated with a small chocolate cupcake that my father bought at the hospital canteen. After the first cycle of chemo I had gotten my hair cut short into a bob style, but after the second cycle my hair started falling out at a faster rate and I had to get it cut even shorter. By the end of my chemo treatments, I lost enough hair that my dad decided to get my head shaved bald—after all, I'd be losing those strands of hair anyway. Being bald wasn't fun at first. I was nervous from the very first moment I stepped into the salon, and the sight of the razor going up and down frightened me even more. After the last of my beautiful hair fell down onto the floor around my chair, I refused to look at myself in the mirror. I was feeling pretty depressed when I left the salon and cried a lot the rest of the day.

In the morning, I woke up and felt my head. The skin was especially soft, and hairless; part of me had hoped that losing my hair had just been a dream. I finally took a good look at myself in the mirror. I thought I looked pretty pitiful without any hair, but I knew I had a lot of strength within me. Seeing how upset I was over the loss of my hair, my brother went to Target and bought me a purple cap to wear. That made me feel a bit better. After a little time, I saw that I didn't have to feel ashamed; in the United States, nobody cares what hairstyle you have. I could have walked down the street with my bald head, and no one would judge me for it. Once I realized that, I was able to enjoy being bald. It was like having a fun new hairstyle, and touching my head was a cool feeling, too. The hair that was starting to grow back didn't feel anything like the hair I'd had before but was soft like a baby's, totally new and fresh.

The day after I had my head shaved, I reported to the chemo station for another treatment. I couldn't help remembering a time that I had gotten a bad haircut. The hairdresser had cut it far too short, and I remember I was so embarrassed that I didn't want to go to school. Back then, I actually cried over having to be seen with my bad haircut. In the hospital, though, it was quite common to be bald, especially in the chemo station. My nurses even gave me compliments on my new purple headwear, which really helped me to feel less self-conscious and more normal. I still put on my cap when I was going outside—the purple cap was now my companion, sitting on my head and watching my every move, wherever I went—but I stopped wearing it when I was indoors. I learned to be proud of being bald.

Whether it was losing my hair, feeling ill from the treatments, or adjusting to the changes in my diet, I always knew I had my family around me to help me through. When I was feeling sick, I almost never left my father's lap; even if I threw up, he took it very lightly and didn't get upset with me at all. I cried often—sometimes it felt like it was a part of my daily routine—but the pain management team at the hospital was incredible and even when I felt bad, I knew the doctors would help me feel better soon. I was very conscious of avoiding junk food and knew I had to respect my treatment. God forbid I have to go through the whole process over again. When I was at the house, I played basketball to stay busy. I enjoyed reading *The Chronicles of Narnia*, which took my mind off of my problems and sent it to a magical world. When I received my treatments at the chemo station, I kept myself entertained playing on my tablet, or using the coloring board. Other times I took the whole chemo machine to the window and sat watching the weather outside. I always kept my stuffed bunny with me—in the hospital, in my bedroom, or riding in my car, it stayed at my side, like my little pet. One time a singer came into the hospital to cheer up the patients. He had his guitar and lyrics on his iPad. He told me that a few years ago, another girl my age was undergoing chemotherapy and he had visited her just like he was visiting me. She also grew up to be a singer, Paige Armstrong, who has released her own album. Watching a live singer was definitely the highlight of the day. My priorities also gradually shifted over the weeks I spent in treatment. When I'd had my surgery back in August, I hated the idea of missing any school, but now that I was in the midst of my chemotherapy, I didn't even want any study material near me. The school did send me notes by email from time to time, but I couldn't ever bring myself to learn them. Even the *Harry Potter* book I'd brought along sat on my shelf unread.

I'm a very outgoing person who enjoys being around people. This was one of the hardest parts about going through the chemotherapy treatments. I couldn't go out in public during busy times because of how badly my immune system was impaired. You never know who around you would have a cold or virus, so there was always a fear of catching an infection if I was out around other people. Abhishek [eldest? yes] helped me to feel less isolated by taking me for a ride in his car at least once a day. He had a very nice car, a brand-new Lexus with a great collection of music to listen to. We would go for long drives at night that sometimes ended at a shopping center—when it was the off-hours of the day, I was sometimes able to go into the shops, since there weren't as many people around that could give me their germs. I especially remember going to a Wegmans that was about five miles from the home where we were staying. Wegmans is an American supermarket chain, and it had a completely different atmosphere from the grocery stores back in India. I especially loved the lighting and would always take a trip through the bakery to stare at all the delicious desserts, even though I was still restricted to healthy foods and couldn't eat them.

It was protocol for the doctors to administer at least three rounds of chemotherapy. By the end of my second cycle my AFP range was down to two digits—a lot lower than it had been when I started. I hoped they would tell me there was no need for the third round, but unfortunately, I would have no choice but to receive it. I told myself at least I only had to have three rounds. Some treatment plans called for six or more; there were some patients who received regular chemotherapy for years. Once I'd finished with my third cycle, I was at least hopeful that I would be done for good.

The first day of my third cycle came on December 18th, 2013. It was a normal enough day, as far as the treatment was concerned, but I was surprised to find myself feeling a bit nostalgic as we finished up for the day. I even cried that evening before leaving my chemo room. I realized I had started enjoying the atmosphere, even if the treatments themselves were often painful. The second day was shorter, with only two major medicines being administered, so we finished up early in the afternoon. To celebrate, my dad took me to the GUESS shop in the Hershey mall and bought me two jackets: one that was bright red, and another that was red leather with a "G" for Guess on the zipper. I didn't like the leather one at first but it started to grow on me the more I looked at it. It was a sophisticated and sober design, if a bit old-fashioned; my dad has always had a great fashion sense.

These jackets weren't the only presents I got to celebrate the end of my third round of chemo. The Pediatric Oncology department gave me a big, soft stuffed bear that could be turned into a pillow. The Never Ever Give Up foundation (or NEGU, for short) gave me a Joy Jar filled with tons of things that could make anyone happy. I also got a basket full of candies and a huge poster from the hospital before I left on the last day of my treatment. I made sure to prepare a "Thank You" card for the hospital and its staff before we went home, extending a warm welcome to India to all of them. The chemo treatments had lasted a lot longer and been a lot harder than recovering from my initial surgery, but I'd also made a lot of happy memories along the way. I was glad it was over but a little sad, too. The end of the treatments meant the return to India—to school, my friends, and the old life I'd been so reluctant to leave behind.

Before we left Pennsylvania, Abbu Bhaiya took me to Hershey's Chocolate World one last time. If you've never heard of it, Hershey's Chocolate World is a chocolate factory that brings together fun rides with delicious treats. I always went to the park whenever I visited Harrisburg, at least partially because they would give the guests free chocolate (although these free chocolates shrunk from a full Hershey bar to a Reese's two pack to a single Hershey Kiss over the time I was going there). On this last visit, my brother and I made a huge cupcake with tons of chocolates and Hershey syrup on top. We also designed our own chocolates, ate a delicious lunch, and went on the tour that showed us how to make chocolates—a tour I must have taken a dozen times before. Even more than the factory itself, I was thrilled just to be out and about among people again. My cancer nightmare seemed to finally be over—reason enough for both me and my brother to celebrate.

Chapter 8

I was lucky in a lot of ways when it came to my chemotherapy treatments. That might sound like an odd thing to hear from someone who's had cancer, but the truth is it could have been so much worse. Especially considering the kind of tumor that I had—how difficult it could be to diagnose, and how rare it typically is for someone my age—I was quite fortunate that I needed only a handful of cycles of the drugs. Only a few months passed between diagnosis and remission. It certainly seemed like longer while it was happening; it was a bit shocking to look back after it was all over and realize how quickly everything had transpired.

I survived; that's the most important thing. I also didn't suffer any complications during my treatment. I was considered an out-patient for treatment purposes since I didn't have to stay in the hospital overnight. A couple of times I had to be rushed back to the hospital because I was feeling too sick or sore, but for the most part I was able to endure the aftermath of the treatments on my own—even if the nights after the drugs were administered could be a bit rough. The nausea and vomiting were the hardest side effects to deal with, and sometimes I would feel so miserable that I would cry, but these symptoms were never too severe. Even when I did need to see the doctors for an unexpected check-up, it was never severe enough to require hospitalization, not even for a few days for observation.

Feeling sick as often as I did made me not want to eat very much. I was served a full dinner the night before I had my surgery at Fortis: cooked paneer, curd, roti, rice, and fresh vegetables like cucumbers, onions, and radishes. At the time I hadn't been very hungry and had eaten only a little of what was served to me. I didn't think about the fact that this would be my last full meal for a while—if I had, I might have forced myself to eat a bit more of what was offered. I was feeling very good at that point, though. Even right before my surgery, when I was already dressed in my hospital clothes and shower cap, I was playing around in my wheelchair and laughing with Sonu bhaiya. I didn't even feel any of the stomach pain that had brought my cancer to the attention of the doctors until right before I was wheeled into the operating theater, and by that point it was just a matter of minutes before the doctors put the IV in my arm to administer my anesthesia and I fell asleep almost instantly, waking up only after the surgery was over.

After my surgery, my stomach pains got even worse. I frequently felt the need to vomit while I was in Fortis recovering. The nurses anticipated this and brought me a steel bowl to be sick in if I needed it, but nothing would come out; it was just a pervasive feeling of nausea. This was disappointing in a way; if I'd been able to throw up, I probably would have felt better, at least for a little bit. Certainly, though, I didn't feel like eating very much, even once enough time had passed that I was allowed to eat solid foods when I wanted to. It was exciting enough for me to get to the point that I could stand up and walk to the bathroom on my own, though the lack of nutrients in my body combined with the trauma from the surgery made me very weak at first. Maybe it was because I was eating so little, or maybe it was caused by the surgery and the medication that was still being administered through my IV, but I was cold all the time when I was in the hospital, even when the visitors sitting in the room with me said they were sweating. I could watch people preparing food and enjoy it—that was how Sonu bhaiya and I spent a lot of our time together, in fact—but even if my mouth was watering for the dishes I saw on TV, I wouldn't have really wanted to eat them if they'd been set in front of me.

Then came the chemotherapy—something else that did nothing to make my stomach feel any better. As small as my appetite had been before, it decreased even more from the chemo medication. There was no need for the doctors to restrict my diet because the medicine took away my desire to eat junk food like pizza and chocolate. Even forcing myself to drink bottles of fruit and vegetable juice was something of a chore. My diet consisted mostly of crackers and Gatorade, especially on the days I went into the hospital to have one of my drug cycles administered. There was one drug in particular that they gave to me to prevent nausea, but it also made me feel very tired and gave me a strange taste in my mouth. I would usually pop a mint, hard candy, or stick of gum into my mouth once they gave me the drug to try and keep myself from tasting it. When I did have a taste for a treat, it was common for me to just get a hot chocolate from Starbucks, or a similar sweet drink, more than it was for me to get myself junk food.

Chemotherapy is such a hard medical procedure to undergo because the drugs administered during it are harmful to living cells. This is why they're effective treatments for cancer. They kill off the cancer cells in short order—and many of the body's healthy cells as collateral damage. Even though I waited the recommended six weeks after the surgery to start my chemotherapy treatments, I wasn't completely back to full strength when they began. At least, it didn't feel like I had made as much progress as I should have in that time. When I was released from Fortis Hospital, for example, I was feeling strong enough that I wanted to walk from my room to the exit instead of taking the wheelchair they'd brought for me. My strength gradually came back over the weeks of recovery before the treatments, but once I began going through the chemo I felt weak again and often didn't want to do anything except sleep.

My last chemotherapy treatment took place in December of 2013. We didn't linger long once the procedure was finished. As soon as I'd had my blood tested for the cancer markers and was given a clean bill of health by the doctors at Hershey, my dad began to make our travel plans to return to India. We flew back to our hometown in January of 2014, a mere month after I was finished with my treatment. I was excited to return to my hometown—more so than I'd been after my previous visits to the United States, though that made sense, given the reason that had brought us to the country on this particular trip. Even though this stay had been just a matter of months as opposed to the two years my dad and I lived in the United States when he was teaching there, it felt like we'd been away for a very long time.

This was especially true when it came to school. I had been trying to keep up with my studies as much as I could on my own, but my focus had been mainly on my treatment and recovery. I'd barely thought about schoolwork at all during my time at Hershey. Since being told I'd be returning to India I picked up the books again, and had been studying about an hour every day between the end of my chemo and my return to classes. When I got back to India I resumed study sessions for math and science with my old tutor, Ms. Vinita, to prepare me to go back to school and pick up where I'd left off. My hair still hadn't grown back and that made me a little bit embarrassed and nervous about how the other kids would react. I was proud to show off my colorful head-gear, though, and liked that it made me look unique from the others in my school.

I'd been a bit nervous that I would fall behind in school from missing so much time. Right around the time of my surgery I had been scheduled to take my 1st-term exams. I still hadn't had a chance to make those up, but the 2nd-term exams for my year were already coming up in the very near future—only a month or so after my return to India. Before the exams, I visited my best friend, Muskaan Bhasin, so I could make copies of her notes and assignments. I knew she kept them neat and in order, much better than most of my classmates. I figured this would make her an excellent person to get the information from if I wanted to have the best chance of performing well on the tests.

Going to Muskaan's house was the first time I saw one of my old friends since I came back and I was a bit apprehensive about it. I felt strange wearing my purple cap over my hairless scalp, but Muskaan acted like everything was normal and that set me at ease. When I arrived, she got me a glass of water and gave me some letters my classmates had written wishing me good health and a speedy recovery. I had planned to just take the notes and go, but she had such a positive vibe and we were having such a good time talking that I stayed for a bit, happy to be sharing time with my friends again.

Between the surgery and the chemotherapy treatments, I had missed six whole months of school. My return coincided exactly with the first day of exams. I had butterflies in my stomach like it was my first day of school. I wasn't sure if I was ready to take my tests. I had spent a lot of time studying recently, but I didn't know if that would be enough to get me caught up with all of the time I had missed. I was also not sure if I would feel the same excitement about school that I had felt before my surgery. I had a different perspective on things now. I wasn't sure if school would feel as important.

It was funny thinking back to when I'd been recovering at Fortis Hospital. I had felt so anxious about missing my 1st term exams when I was preparing for surgery. I remember how happy I'd been to see my teachers, Ms. Supriti Bhadra and Ms. Sapna Gajwani, when they'd stopped by to visit me a few days after my surgery. Before I went to the hospital, my school chess team won a silver medal in chess in an inter-school competition throughout Chandigarh. The teachers had come to give me my medal, hanging it on one of the hooks of my IV rack so that I could see it and feel proud of my accomplishment. They'd wished me fast healing and admonished me, as my father had, not to worry at all about my studies or feel any pressure to rush back to them. Seeing them had practically brought tears to my eyes and I'd been filled with nostalgia after they left, already longing for the return of my school days. Now that the time for that return had come, though, my feelings had shifted.

I would be going back to the same classroom I'd had before, would be instructed by the same teacher. The reason things felt different was because of the ways that I had changed. I wasn't sure how much that would affect me once I saw my friends and started going back to classes. I wore my favorite purple cap to give me strength. Just like with going to Muskaan's for the notes, it turned out there was no reason for me to worry. Muskaan, Damini, and my other friends had decorated the classroom to show how excited they were to have me back. I was dumbstruck by the display. The walls were covered with colorful balloons, strings, and banners. It felt like it was my birthday. Everyone in the class smiled and greeted me happily. They showered me with get well soon cards they'd made themselves. I truly felt like I had been welcomed home.

Once we took our seats, celebration time was over. It was time for us to begin our tests. I did some quick last-minute reviewing, even though I knew I was prepared. As the test started, though, I realized I wasn't as nervous as I thought I would've been—certainly not as anxious as I'd been at the thought of missing my 1st term exams the previous August. The cancer treatments had truly brought me a new outlook on everything. The test was important, certainly, but it wasn't nearly as important as my health. It made it easier to simply take the test and not worry about the outcome when I knew it wasn't as serious.

As it turned out, I didn't need to worry about the tests anyway. I was better prepared for them than I realized. I passed my 8th grade exams with flying colors: a 64 in Hindi, a 70 in French, over 80 in English, Science, and Social Science, and over 90 in Math. Not only did I get high scores, I even received a scholar badge. It was good to get back into the swing of things and feel like my life was getting back to normal. With my exams completed, I moved up to 9th grade with the rest of my classmates. It was as if I had never missed any time in school at all.

I wasn't feeling pain or discomfort from either my illness or the treatment anymore by this point. Even so, my medical team from back in Hershey had a detailed regime of follow-up health checks they wanted me to undergo occasionally. There wasn't any trace of cancer left in my system when I'd finished my chemotherapy, but that wasn't a guarantee that the disease would never reoccur. What had happened to my mother was a vivid reminder of this fact. This is why people referred to cancer as being in remission rather than being cured; there is always a lingering threat of re-occurrence, and the few years immediately following my treatment were the riskiest time as far as this was concerned.

The tests recommended by Hershey included blood tests to check for tumor markers, MRI scans, chest x-rays, and audiology reports, all of which were to be administered on the schedule they'd outlined. The letter detailing all of this information arrived a bit later than it was supposed to, so I ended up missing a couple of the recommended tests, but this ended up not being a problem. We set up an appointment to get the tests taken as soon as we did have information about them. The results were positive when we got them back. My AFP levels were continuing to decline, making more progress with each test. Just one good result didn't necessarily mean I was home free. It was recommended that I continue to get the tests taken at least once a year for the next five years. As a precaution, since there was a history of cancer in my family, Dr. Sarla recommended that I instead have my blood tested every three months, with an ultrasound of my mid-section taking place every six months; the rest of the tests I could have done on a yearly basis. I was glad that we had Dr. Sarla around as a resource to keep an eye on my health. Both my dad and I knew that we could trust her recommendations about my health, and that I could call her any time I was feeling any pain to make sure that it wasn't anything serious.

Since everything was going well with me physically, I was able to rejoin my kathak dance class. This was very exciting for me since dancing was one of the things I had really enjoyed doing before, both when I lived in India and while I was living in the United States. I also resumed a lot of other activities that I'd done before my treatments started. I was getting more and more interested in French and started attending formal lessons in the language at a place called Alliance Française.

I also re-joined the morning basketball class with my friend Damini. I had been in the class with her at the start of my 8th grade year and very much enjoyed playing the sport. It was only the onslaught of cancer that had stopped me from continuing to play. This meant my school day would start earlier than it had before. We would begin the class at 6:30am so we could be finished in time to go about the rest of our school day. There were other students who would be there, too, playing other sports like football or tennis, and they weren't all from the 9th grade year. The basketball class itself was a combination of different years of students, everyone from 8th grade to 10th grade playing together. There were about twenty students in the class all told, with both the boys and the girls playing together.

We did a lot more than just play basketball in the morning sports class, too. Our coach, Tejinder Sir, also had us work on our overall health and conditioning. This started with us running around the boundaries of the sporting grounds, usually between four and five times. It didn't look very hard to run around the area but when we were taking that many laps it added up to a pretty long distance, or at least it felt that way that early in the morning. Sometimes we would cheat a little bit by running across the field diagonally from corner to corner when Tejinder Sir wasn't watching us. Even when we cheated like this, though, we would all be pretty exhausted by the time we were done with our rounds. And that was just the start of the practice. After we were done running, we would do our stretching and warming up, often followed by short races between the students on the team across the basketball court.

Finally, we would reach the part of the practice that was specific to the sport. We'd practice shooting lay-ups and long balls, work on defensive moves like rebounds, and of course try to perfect our dribbling and passing. After we'd worked on these kinds of technical skills we would split up into the boys and the girls and play half-court matches. I wasn't a particularly strong player so I usually didn't end up having the ball passed to me very much during the games. We'd finish off the sessions with more stretching, to help keep us from getting sore while we were sitting in school. Even though I wasn't particularly active during the games themselves I always very much enjoyed the entire hour that we spent in morning sports. When it was over, we'd change out of our athletic clothes and back into our school uniforms, starting our school days a little bit before eight in the morning.

It felt good to be able to go back to doing all the same activities I'd been involved in before the onset of cancer. Best of all, I was living a healthy life without having to take any medicine. Even though I was feeling worlds better, I made it a point to pay more attention to my health than I did before I found out about the disease. This was especially true when it came to the kinds of foods I would eat. I'd never really been a health-conscious person before but now I made a point to balance fast food and junk food with healthier meals. Sweet amla murabba became one of my favorite healthy snacks. My dad would also prepare ayurvedic treatments for me. I would start every morning with almond paste and a glass of warm honey water. At night, he would make me a blend of herbs to take, including ginger, garlic, and cardamom, mixed together with honey, raisins, and figs. The taste of raw garlic was a bit difficult to swallow at first but eventually I got used to it. Drinking water with the garlic made it easier to eat.

Most of the stories you hear about cancer and recovery are unhappy accounts of pain and suffering. There were certainly moments after the surgery and during chemotherapy that weren't comfortable, but I often find I have a big smile on my face when I tell people about my cancer and treatment. It was a positive experience overall, and I truly feel like it brought out the best in me. I live better than I did before, and am stronger than I was thanks to having gone through that experience.

One of the biggest physical changes I noticed right away was to my appetite. I had never wanted to eat very much before, or to eat foods that were especially good for me. My dad used to say I would eat like a sparrow. A normal meal for me was half a roti with a bit of lentils or vegetables, and sometimes a piece of fruit as a snack. After the treatments, fruits and vegetables of all kinds looked appealing to me, even ones I hadn't wanted to eat before.

I was hungry much more often than I used to be, too. Thanks to my dad's advice and the knowledge I'd picked up during the treatments, I understood the importance of eating right to maintain my overall good health. I made more of an effort to eat three square meals every day. On school days this was a bit tricky since I had to be there so early for basketball practice and I didn't want to feel too full when I was about to be running around. I would still make sure to eat something, though—usually a banana and some milk along with my morning lemon water. The days I didn't go to school I would make it a point to eat a very hearty breakfast: a prantha or two with curd, or a vegetable omelet on the days my dad felt like cooking.

By lunch time, I would be hungry again. At school, we had a lunch monitor, usually a fellow student from our class that would walk around the cafeteria to make sure everyone finished their meal. Before the cancer, I would almost never finish my food and would have to make an excuse to the lunch monitor to explain why—that I felt full, or had a stomach ache, or something of that nature—then would give my leftovers to my dad to eat when he got home from work. A lot of times, knowing that I wouldn't eat very much, my dad would only make me a small sandwich, one with dal and lentils, or with cauliflower and other vegetables, on slices of brown bread. Even though it was relatively little food, I still usually wouldn't finish it. Once I got back to school in 2014, on the other hand, I had no problem finishing whatever food I'd been given for lunch. Even if there were two pranthas or vegetable rice, or if my dad sent along sweet pancakes with fennel seeds, I would eat every bite.

When it comes to snacking, I've also made some changes. I was never really a huge junk food lover, but when I did snack I would eat some kind of unhealthy treat like ice cream, chocolate, or chips. Now I make a point of eating healthy foods at snack times. One of my favorite new snack choices was to make myself home-squeezed juices in various flavor combinations. I loved the taste of pomegranate juice, especially. It wasn't as if I deprived myself; my dad, Seema and I still went out to eat nice dinner about once a week, and I still ate things like ice cream on occasions, but it was as though I'd lost most of my taste for it.

My dietary habits weren't the only thing that had changed as a result of my experience. I noticed even when I was preparing to go back to school that my priorities had shifted. I wasn't nearly as concerned about school as I had been before. I still knew it was important and wanted to do well, but I wasn't as interested in studying. I didn't take as much time as I used to each day doing my homework, and my scholastic productivity dropped off quite a bit.

What was funny was that it hardly seemed to affect my performance at all. I maintained my usual good marks as I continued with the year, my grades consistently in the top five within my class of about 40 students. I mentioned this to Abhishek and he told me I wasn't alone in this. He and Abhinav had been the same way, at least up through the end of high school. He warned me, though, that this wouldn't carry me through once I got into college. At that point, I would need to work hard if I wanted to continue my success. After having that talk with my brother, I tried to restore some of my motivation, and maintained a habit of reading every night. I'm trying to find the right balance between working hard at my studies and maintaining my good health. I always make a point of staying hydrated and drinking plenty of water throughout the day when I'm studying.

Having cancer changed me for the better. I used to overload my schedule with all kinds of extra-curricular activities and tutoring sessions, going from morning until night and hardly letting myself stop to rest. My dad used to warn me that I shouldn't over-exert myself but I would never listen. I always wanted to push myself harder and do as many things as I could. Now, I paid attention to my body and stopped when I was tired and needed a break. Being able to take things at a bit of a slower pace made it possible for me to focus more on my health.

It also felt like I was more confident in myself. I was better able to accept myself the way I am. After all, I'd survived cancer; I must be pretty strong. All my friends at school noticed I was much more outgoing now than I'd been before. It made it easier not to take negative comments too seriously and appreciate things for what they are. I liked this better version of me and I was ready to keep moving ahead and see what the next year would have in store for me.

Chapter 9

Even though the cancer treatments only lasted for six months, it took a while until I felt I was completely readjusted back to something that felt like normalcy. My 8th grade section was split up when we all started into 9th grade, so at least everyone else was also starting fresh with the new year. My class teacher was Sapna Bhasin, our computers teacher. She's a sweet woman and helped me feel more comfortable as I transitioned back into regular school life.

I thought people would tease me about my cap, but no one did. All of the teachers and the students were very friendly, even the ones I didn't know from before. My hair was starting to grow back underneath it, but it was still much shorter than it had been before my treatment. I kept wearing my cap until my hair was past my ears, around the middle of my 9th grade year.

Starting 9th grade, we had a choice between studying Hindi or French as our second language. Since I already had some background in French, I decided to continue on with my studies of it. Now that I had passed my 2nd term exams and felt like I was caught back up scholastically, I decided to stop going to the tutor. I also had fallen out of the habit of studying, though. I was surprised when my test grades fell dramatically. I was used to being close to the top of my class, so I knew I had to start paying more attention to my studies and buckle down to get my scores back up. My health was important, and I didn't want to overload myself or stress myself out, but I realized I needed to strike a better balance and devote more time and concentration to my school work.

My 9th grade year was quite hectic and exhausting. I would go in early for basketball. Classes started around 7:40 AM and were supposed to run until 2:20 in the afternoon. This time was divided into nine different time slots, each of which was reserved for a different subject, with a different teacher for each. My dad was concerned about my food intake since the only time that I could eat was lunch, which was around 11 AM.

He wrote a letter to the school asking permission for me to leave school at 1:30 PM instead, before the last period of the day. After I got home, I would talk to my friends from my class to find out what had been taught during that last period that I missed.

By the end of my 9th grade year, my marks were back to where they should be. I passed the year with flying colors, ready to move on to the next level. By the time my 10th grade year started, my hair was almost shoulder length. I had a new class teacher, Oorja Mam, who had been my French teacher in 9th grade. I had the same basic schedule as I had the year before and was still allowed to leave at 1:30 PM instead of the usual time.

We were given a project for French class during the 10th grade summer vacation. The assignment was for us to videotape ourselves interviewing each other, on a topic of our choice. I paired up with my friend Damini for the project. We wrote the transcript for the interview together and showed it to Oorja Mam before the vacation started. During the break, we made the video in the park out front of our school building, edited the video together, and sent it along to the teacher.

The school also hosted a French Day after summer vacation. Both the 9th grade and 10th grade French classes participated, decorating the seminar room where it was being held and bringing in delicious home-made food for us to eat. I joined up with my friends Damini, Arshiya, Sharone, and Angel to sing the French song "La vie en Rose" for the class. Instead of wearing our usual school uniforms, we put on dresses that were blue, white, and red, like the French flag. A lot of the school's teachers were there to watch us, both those in the French faculty and teachers from other departments.

I had thought the videos we made over the summer were just for Oorja Mam to test our French fluency, but it turned out there was a larger purpose in mind for them. There was a projector set up at French Day and everyone in attendance watched all of the videos. I saw that many of the students had made them in each other's homes instead of outside. Maybe a smart idea, I realized watching mine and Damani's; the noise of the kids playing in the park made it difficult to hear what we were saying. Despite these little problems, French Day was still a success overall.

I had a lot of fun with my other extracurricular activities during my 10th-grade year, as well. I got the opportunity to dance on stage in the Tagore Theater, during the dance performance Pracheen Kala Kendra organizes every year. I was also still playing chess with my school's team, along with the morning basketball practices—a pretty full schedule, all things considered, though I was careful not to give myself more to do than I could handle.

In April of 2015 there was a chess competition in Chandigarh. It would determine who were the best players in the region, the ones who would be representing the city in the national tournament. I had done well during my matches to that point, winning all of them except for one, which ended in a draw. I mostly played with black, which gave me an edge and led to me being selected as the captain of the team.

The competition was being held in Salem, a city in the district of the same name in the state of Tamil Nadu, about halfway between Coimbatore and Bangalore. We weren't sure what the accommodations would be like for the team so my dad wrote a letter to DPS Chandigarh asking the event's organizers if we would be allowed to arrange our own lodgings. Once they gave approval my dad made all the bookings. We picked up the team's sports kits from a government school in Chandigarh, which included shoes, a track suit, and a bag for each of us.

My dad had to stay behind and finish up some work he had to do for cases in the High Court. He'd be joining us in Salem, but for the initial trip Seema accompanied me instead. We flew from Chandigarh to Bangalore, where we would be staying for the night before continuing on the rest of the way to Salem by bus. When we reached the hotel, we were a bit nervous about the location; it was in a very crowded, urban neighborhood. South India is generally safe, though, and the culture encourages respect for women, so we decided to at least go inside and see what the rooms were like before we looked for alternate accommodations. We were glad we did; when we got upstairs and saw where we'd be staying we were impressed. As an extra bonus, breakfast was complementary. And it wasn't skimpy, either, we found out the next morning. There were a plethora of South Indian dishes put out in banquet serving trays for guests, including idli, vada, sambhar, and chutney, with delicious coffee served after the meal. This was perfect for me since I'm a big fan of South Indian cuisine. There's a restaurant called Sagar Ratna in Chandigarh that serves South Indian food and it was one of my favorite places to go for lunch or dinner.

After breakfast, we packed our bags and went outside to catch an auto-rickshaw to the bus stop. When we got there, we found out we'd tarried too long at our meal; the bus had already gone. Luckily we were able to have the bus authority call ahead and hold our bus at a stop further along the route. The driving in Bangalore is crazier than it is in Delhi, but we reached the bus stop safely and saw other passengers from the area were still boarding the bus. We showed our tickets and got on without a hassle.

The bus was incredible compared to others I'd been on. There was Wi-Fi and air conditioning and the seats were comfortable, with screens showing a movie in front of the seats. It made the four-hour journey to Salem much more comfortable. Even though there were plenty of entertainment options available I spent a lot of the trip just relaxing and staring out the window at the beautiful scenery. It reminded me of taking road trips down the highways in the United States.

When we arrived at the bus station in Salem there was a car waiting to take us to the government rest house where we'd be staying during the competition. We had the car for the entire day so we decided to take a little drive to the school where they'd be holding the competition. When we looked at the directions to get there, though, we saw it was quite far away and decided not to take the trip after all. Instead, we looked for a place to eat lunch. We were hoping to find a nice restaurant but there was nothing in the area of our hotel. We ate Domino's instead, going for convenience. My dad got in pretty late at night and we settled in to get rest and prepare for the next day.

The next day we met our driver and tour guide, Mr. Balu, a wonderful and knowledgeable man who would be with us for the rest of our trip. I had already proudly donned my team track suit with "Chandigarh" written on the back. Mr. Balu drove us to the contest site in time for us to eat some breakfast. They'd arranged for the competitors to have a basic breakfast of eggs, bread, and such, but there were also a lot of food stalls in the area so Seema and I decided to get breakfast from there. We checked in quickly, receiving identification cards. Soon after that, the tournament began.

There were quite a few states from India competing—it was definitely the largest chess tournament I'd ever played in. Each player was given a notebook to record their moves. We were playing timed games, as well. Every player was given a certain amount of time on the clock to make their moves and had to finish the game before that time ran out. If they didn't, the player who ran out of time first would lose. After a long first day of playing, we stopped back at the hotel before dinner. Mr. Balu took us to a wonderful fine dining restaurant. We had a delicious meal of lentils and Indian bread with some nicely-cooked potato and cauliflower.

The second day started much the same as the first had. During the tournament, though, one of the players from my school fell sick. We'd brought along an extra player, who now jumped in and took their place. As the captain, I had to fill out the necessary paperwork to make the change. I hadn't realized before that my position involved more than motivating the team.

We did a bit of sight-seeing after the second day of competition. Mr. Balu drove us up to a temple built into a steep hillside. The road leading up to it was full of hair-pin turns—frightening to ride down, though our driver handled them with ease. The sight from the top was certainly worth the drive up. The temple itself was beautiful, filled with lighted candles, the air perfumed by incense. We also went to a Hanuman temple and a Shiv temple during our trip. The Shiv temple was especially magnificent. There was a lovely calm environment around it, and we even saw an elephant while we were there. Along with the places we visited, I greatly enjoyed the various restaurants we ate at, even the ones that were more fast food than fine dining. There was one chain we ate at often that I remember vividly: Hotel Saravana Bhavan, a South Indian restaurant chain and one of the largest vegetarian restaurant chains in the world. They served a dish called idli-upama that was difficult to find in Northern India.

With so many great teams to compete against, my school didn't place very high in the competition. None of us were particularly disappointed by this, though. The trip wasn't about winning; it was about enjoying the experience and getting to play against and learn from a wide array of different players. At the very least it was a nice little break from the school routine back home in Chandigarh.

As my 10th grade year was nearing its end, I got a call from Oorja Mam asking me to come into the school. When I got there, she asked if I could send her a photo and a brief passage about me. I wasn't sure why she would need this information. I knew the 2nd-term exam results were going to be announced soon, so I had my dad check them online using my roll number. Much to the surprise of both me and my father, we learned I'd received a 10 CGPA. I had to see the result for myself on his laptop screen before I believed it. While I'd been studying more than when I first returned to school, I didn't think I had put in enough effort to obtain perfect results. I was thrilled and raced off to the school.

There were about a dozen students who'd received perfect results on their exams. Media people came in to interview us. As we were hopping onto the bus to take us home, a drone was circling the air snapping pictures. Along with the congratulations for the high scores themselves, the teachers had picked out the names of those students who scored well despite having encountered many obstacles. My name was given, along with another classmate, Naumika, who suffers from both epilepsy and diabetes.

After these score announcements were made, I was contacted by writers from various local newspapers asking me to share the story of my cancer treatment and survival. Quite a few newspapers ran articles or passages about me the next day. This was the first time I had ever been written about in a newspaper, and I was pretty excited about it. I received calls from a lot of my friends giving me congratulations. It was pretty nice to feel like I was famous for a little while.

With grade 10 over, it was time to move up to grade 11. The school day ended at 1 PM for students in grades 11 and 12 at DPS Chandigarh, which meant I didn't have to miss the last class of the day anymore. I had pretty high standards to uphold now, having received a perfect score on my last exams, and I knew expectations for me would be high, but that had never bothered me before.

I continued to play chess and compete in tournaments when I was able. In May of my 11th-grade year, the Under-17 girls' team traveled to Surat to play in the Inter-DPS National Tournament. Two players were selected to go from each school. I was one of the players for my school, along with Ishita Arora. We tried to make our own arrangements for accommodations, just like we had for the tournament in Salem, but DPS Surat insisted they had top-tier facilities and all of the competing students were required to stay where the school had arranged. My dad still made separate arrangements for me to get to Surat, again with Seema accompanying me, while Ishita and our supervising teacher, Sharmita Mam, went on their own.

It was another multi-stage journey to get to Surat. We flew from Chandigarh Airport to Mumbai. My dad had family living there, a younger cousin, Mr. Madan who offered to let us stay with him for the night. He sent a car to pick us up from the airport. When we reached his house, his wife Mrs. Minnie gave us a warm welcome. We put our things down in the room where we'd be sleeping then sat with her, chatting and drinking refreshing sweet lassi. They had an elaborately decorated chess board, much more so than the sets I was used to playing on. It was a bit difficult to tell what the pieces were. Once I figured everything out and put some concentration into it, I started winning the games.

After eating the delicious dinner Minnie aunty made for us, we took a trip to a nearby beach to relax for the evening. There was a stand serving kala khatta, a dessert that's like a popsicle dipped in a sweet and sour, cola-flavored syrup. It was the perfect way to finish off our evening.

The next morning, Madan uncle took us to catch our train the rest of the way from Mumbai to Surat. It was a long trip, nearly five hours, but the seats on the train were so comfortable I had no trouble settling in, and I was well-rested, having gotten good sleep the night before. Just like on the bus trip the last spring, I spent most of the journey looking out the window, watching the scenery pass by.

When we reached Surat, an auto-rickshaw took us straight up to the school. I was pretty amazed by how big it was when we went inside. There were large halls where the mattresses had been laid out for the participants, about ten beds in each, all of them made up with covers provided by the host school. A lot of students had arrived already from various schools around the country. Seema and I met up with Ishita and Sharmita Mam then mingled with the other kids. Everyone was so friendly that we had a great time hanging out with them. The food in the dining area was pretty good, too. We found that out at dinner that first night and it held true for every meal, and the snacks in between.

We were supposed to be in our beds and asleep by 10:30 so that we could get a good night's rest and be fresh and alert for the competition. The next morning we woke up early, had breakfast, and made our way to the building where the tournament would take place, which was just across from the one we were staying in. The teams all took an oath to follow all the rules and regulations and not cheat, under any circumstances. The host school held a cultural program in the same room where we would be playing. Once the program was over, all of the participants stood for the playing of the national anthem. After it, the Principal went on-stage and gave a short speech, encouraging all the participants to play to the best of our abilities. It was an excellent speech, concise and to the point while still being very motivating. I didn't feel bored even once during the Principal's speech, and that was pretty surprising—most speeches I've had to sit through, my mind started to wander by the end.

Once we'd completed all the inaugural ceremonies, the competition got started. There were so many matches that I can't remember how many our team even won. To tell the truth, the other things we did while we were in Surat stand out more in my mind than the tournament itself. There were a lot of other games besides chess that we could play. The school's tennis and basketball courts were adjacent to the competition building. There was also a large indoor gym with table tennis and badminton. Not only were we allowed to use these facilities, the school's coaches for each game were on-hand to give us tips and help us play the different games. We could swim in the school's pool at night under the supervision of the swimming coach. They didn't even demand that we wore a bathing suit. One night, I jumped into the pool in my regular clothes one night, then just changed into a different outfit afterwards for the rest of the evening. They also let us plug our phones into the PA system in the basketball courts at night, so a few of the participants had an impromptu dance party.

One of the evenings of the tournament we were paid a visit by Vikramaditya Kulkarni, an internationally-renowned chess master. He was such a skilled player that he could keep track of multiple games at the same time. To demonstrate this, he instructed all of the tournament players to sit in a big circle. He made his way around the circle, stopping at each board and moving a piece. Obviously none of us were able to beat him, but we all wrote down his moves so we could study them more closely during our free time. It was a good experience getting to play against such an experienced player.

The second night of the tournament the host school's music faculty put on a performance for the participants and their teachers. They were all very skilled and their performance was enjoyable to listen to, but that wasn't even the most fun part of the evening. Once the officially scheduled performance was over, they asked the members of the audience if anyone wanted to perform. Any students who wanted to sing were given the mic. A lot of them had really good singing voices. Since Sharmita Mam knew about my background in dance, she asked me to get up and show everyone some of my kathak moves. She brought up "Tarana in Raag Kalavati" on YouTube on her phone then attached it to the speakers as a background for my performance. I hadn't expected to be putting on a performance, and I was a bit nervous when I started about dancing solo in front of everyone. At the end everybody clapped in appreciation for my performance and I was happy I'd had the nerve to get up and do it.

When we were getting ready for sleep after the cultural performance, I noticed the underside of my foot was swollen and bruised. I realized the rough surface of the basketball court had injured my foot. Kathak is danced barefoot to give the steps the most percussive sound, but not normally on a surface that hard. The contusion healed by the end of the week, thankfully, though it felt a bit sore to walk on for a couple of days.

We visited an aquarium the next day. It was further away than the other activities we'd done so far, about a thirty-minute drive from the school. When we'd had our fill of looking at the sea creatures, we visited an amazing temple nearby. Back at the school we practiced a few chess games and ate dinner before going to sleep. The sun rose bright and shining the next day. Some of the teams—teachers as well as students—went out shopping at markets nearby. Seema and I visited a wholesale market and she bought some cloth she planned to take back to Chandigarh to get stitched.

I was definitely sad to leave Surat. The host school had been so incredibly hospitable, and it had been a much better experience overall than the previous year's tournament in Salem—not that the first tournament was bad, either; the one in Surat was just especially fun. Every school that participated received a small trophy shaped like a pawn, regardless of where they ended up in the standings.

On the way back to Chandigarh, we again stayed with Madan uncle in Mumbai. We decided to continue our sight-seeing and woke up early the next morning—around 6 AM—to catch a taxi into the city. We had it drop us off at the Gateway of India in Colaba. It was a blustery day, the air fresh with the smell of the sea. Birds were circling in the morning air. It was an idyllic scene. We walked around for a bit, enjoying a light snack of bananas and coconut before we called the taxi back to take us home.

There was a delicious ice cream parlor in Mumbai. Minnie aunty had served us some for dessert the night before. Because we'd loved it so much, she ordered some for us to take with us back to Chandigarh. I was dubious about how we would be able to transport the ice cream on the plane, but it was apparently not as unusual as I would've thought. They had a special bag that kept the ice cream packed in dry ice, preventing it from melting even if it was out of the freezer for a long time. It was certainly worth the effort. I'm pretty sure it was the most flavorful and natural-tasting ice cream I've ever had, and it came in so many fantastic flavors, like coconut, sapodilla, and mango. My dad picked us up at the airport when our flight landed. The first thing I did when he got us home was open up the ice cream—that's just how delicious it was.

Along with my travels around India, my dad and I went back to Pennsylvania to visit in the summer of 2016. The most fascinating thing we did on this trip was visit an Amish village. The Amish are a religious group that's based mostly in the United States, although settlements have spread into Canada. Visiting their region made me think of the traditional villages we have in India, although perhaps a bit more civilized. Our tour of the village lasted about ninety minutes, during which time the tour guide explained the details of Amish culture. Their schooling was very different than other places in the United States. Each school would provide education for the kids who lived within about five kilometers and everyone would attend school together, no matter how old they were. Amish kids also didn't go through as much schooling as other kids, attending classes only through the 8th grade before they would begin helping their families on the farms full-time.

Maybe the best-known feature of Amish culture is the fact that they're not allowed to use electricity. They still navigate in horse-drawn carriages instead of cars and use oil lamps and other non-electric lighting. They are also highly self-sufficient. Amish societies raise all of their own food and make all of their own clothes, which are simple in design, mostly solid colors with no buttons, jewelry, or adornments. Their society is very insular on the whole. Amish people are only allowed to marry other Amish, a system known as endogamy. If someone who was raised Amish wants to move to a city, marry someone outside the community, get higher education—anything that doesn't happen within the community, basically—they're allowed to, but they are no longer considered Amish once they do, and have to move away from the community.

Since my dad comes from a legal background, he was very curious how the Amish legal system worked. The tour guide explained that all disputes are settled within the family, rather than in official courts. Many of the things other cultures need lawyers for weren't even issues within Amish culture. There was no divorce, for example, and much more communal than personal property. By the time we were done with the tour, I had concluded that Amish society was interesting but I would definitely not want to live in it.

Between all my trips and activities, my high school years moved so fast. Before I knew it, they were nearly over. After that quick drop at the beginning, my grades had remained at their usual high standard throughout my high school years. During my 12th grade year, my father got a call from Mr. Mishra, telling him I was one of ten students in our tri-city area selected for a prestigious award. Mr. Mishra had established a charitable trust in his father's name, and was an organizer of various charity events honoring and encouraging women and children from the region. I was to be honored at the Beti Samaan Samaroah, an event honoring talented girls. I thought at first that it might have been a hoax call since it came completely out of the blue, but my father had heard of it before. Abhinav had also received the award when he was in school.

On the date of the award ceremony, we went to Manav Mangali Smart School in Mohali and were met by Mr. Mishra at the entrance. He guided us to the auditorium where the event was set to take place. I didn't really believe I was going to receive the award until I actually reached the hall and saw several of the other award recipients sitting there with their parents. The audience for the event was made up of students from the Manav Mangali Smart School. Some of the students also put on a musical to kick off the ceremony. It was focused on the achievements of women across occupations. It was very inspiring and well-performed, an excellent introduction to the day's events.

When it came time to honor the award recipients, I happened to be called first. I walked across the stage with a lump in my throat, receiving my award from the governor to the accompaniment of camera clicks from the reporters in the audience. Since I was the first, I ended up standing on the other side of the stage by myself while the next recipient was honored. She was a young blind girl with a great talent for oration. After she was introduced and received her award, she gave a short acceptance speech on the power of women. You could hear a pin drop in the hall after she'd finished. Everyone in the audience was entranced by her bravery and powerful words.

The rest of the award winners were honored then, all of us remaining on the stage until they'd taken the final group photograph. With that done, we took our seats to listen to the Governor give a speech. The award wasn't just for points of pride. It came with a cash prize: 10,000 rupees for each child along with a significant donation for the school. The event was delightful and unforgettable, and it was exciting to again see myself in the newspaper the next day; every local paper had some kind of article about the event.

The harrowing ordeal that was my cancer treatments, by now, seemed far in the past. My health hadn't faltered since our return to India. I was still receiving regular check-ups to make sure the cancer hadn't returned, and they consistently came back clean. While I now understood, better than I had before, that lifelong health was a lifelong commitment, I knew I could maintain it and make great strides and achievements in my life. I had found my balance between health and productivity. As I finished with my secondary schooling, I knew this would continue to lead me to great things in the future.

Chapter 10

It has been 6 years since my cancer tumor was removed. By now, the regular cancer treatments and check-up regiment is over. At my last check, there were no traces of the disease, and while I know there is always the chance of a relapse, the cancer seems to be a thing of the past. I take pride in being a cancer survivor. Having gone through such a trial at such a young age seems to make my weaknesses in other areas seem less important. My academic performance, social interactions, involvement in extra-curricular activities—none of these are as important as life. No matter how I do in any of those areas, it cannot change the fact that I fought cancer and prevailed.

It is not entirely correct to say that my cancer has been treated. Rather, I should think of it as being in long-term remission, because—as my dad reminds me from time to time—it can come back at any point. This was the mistake my mom made. She thought her health was in the clear, then was blindsided by a disease relapse. Keeping this possibility in mind helps me stay aware of my health and do everything I can to keep the cancer from returning, yet enjoy life at the same time. I've improved my eating habits, make sure to get plenty of exercise, stay aware of the conditions of my surroundings and environment, and overall strive to maintain a healthy lifestyle. I know by making these little changes I can help keep my health strong for many years to come—can continue to live my life, my way.

When I was going through my chemotherapy treatments at Hershey Hospital, I never once thought that my life would be ending soon. It seemed to me instead like a new beginning, or a re-birth. Every day I looked forward more and more to being back in India, greeting all my friends and those dear to me. I just knew I had to get back there, that this wouldn't be the end for me. I missed all the parts of school: making projects, doing homework, studying for my exams the day before and passing them with flying colors—even the aspects of it that most kids would be happy to avoid were things that I enjoyed and was eager to get back to. I woke up each morning excited to start a new day. This, I think, was part of why I was able to recover so fully. I continued to look forward, staying strong on the inside even when my body was weak, and this strength helped me to push through; I always know there is some external energy which continuously gives me power to face any circumstance that might come.

I owe much of this outlook on my future, as well as my current good health, to my dad, my brother, all of my well-wishers, and the team of doctors who took care of me during my treatment. I have kept in touch with many of the doctors who aided in my recovery. I still see Dr. Sarla and Dr. Wig in a social context from time to time. I have also gone back to the Hershey area and visited the doctors and nurses since my return to India. The staff at Hershey Hospital has changed quite a bit since I was undergoing my treatment there. On my most recent visit, Dr. Shivani Shah and Dr. Fecile had both left Hershey, and I could find only one of the Pediatric Oncology Center nurses I had worked with. She recognized me instantly, though, and was thrilled to see me doing so well.

I'm an ardent student of spirituality. In my continuing journey on this path, I've read many books on Hinduism that were given to me as gifts by Rama Krishna Mission Ashram Chandigarh. My father had previously recounted some stories to me from one of them, *Autobiography of a Yogi* by Parmahansa Yogananda, which is one of the most popular philosophical books. These stories touched me deeply, motivating me to be educated further on the subject. These studies have greatly aided me in expanding my understanding of spirituality, as well as of myself.

I've also been inspired by spiritual leaders from various organizations throughout my journey. They've helped me find the strength to overcome obstacles and stress, no matter how large. Even now, I feel extra motivation when I see the faces of these inspiring leaders and think about the journeys they took in their own lives. During our time on this planet, we should strive to act in ways that are for the good of all people and try to avoid generating bad karma by making decisions and actions that are not harmful to others. Reading books written by eminent spiritual scholars has taught me that life can be simple if you chose to make it. Someone who is easy-going and has peace in their heart will be surrounded constantly by happiness and will be able to overcome any obstacle; if you perceive life as a struggle and project negative energy, that negativity will be returned to you in kind. There is an Indian phrase I like to think of, which goes, "*Man ke hare haar hai, man ke jite jeet.*" This phrase carries roughly the same meaning as what Swami Vivekanand said: "Strength is life, weakness is death." I believe this is true in all parts of life.

Newton's Third Law states that for every action there is an equal and opposite reaction. This is the law of karma, too. Actions that hurt other people bounce back on you, too. When you create a negative environment by even having bad thoughts about a person, it surrounds you with a negative energy. If you instead create a positive aura within yourself and in the ways you interact with others, it dispels those negative energies. It may sound silly to say you can think yourself happy or think yourself well, but there are studies that show people can heal their bodies by controlling their states of mind. Positive thinking can even help to overcome deadly diseases, like cancer. A study conducted by John's Hopkins medical center's Lisa R. Yanek[1] showed that those with a positive outlook on life were less likely to suffer from heart disease as they age, while those with a more negative outlook tend to have a weaker immune response and suffer from more stress-related health issues. The staff of the Mayo Clinic also released a study in recent years about the health benefits of positive self-talk, which can include lowered depression rates, greater germ resistance, and an increased life span. A book I enjoyed reading recently is *The Power of Positive Thinking* by the author Norman Vincent Peale. It is a self-help book which proposes various distinct practical methods to experience the benefits of positive thinking. The long and short of it is that, although then body and mind are separate, their working condition has a direct impact on each other.

I am as careful now about controlling my energy and maintaining a positive state of mind as I am about my physical nutrition and health. If I stay happy, I will be healthy. That is the ideology I aim to follow. There's no room for sadness if happiness occupies all the space in the heart. When I'm feeling low, I talk to myself. I think about my day: where I went and who I talked to, especially thinking about any negative interactions I had during the day. Thinking through each day lets me purge these disturbed thoughts from my mind and correct any mistakes I made, whether they were with the words I said or the way I said them. If I said something false, I immediately check the facts when I get home so I can speak the truth and back it up the next time the topic comes up. Talking through my days like this also lets me process my thoughts, coming up with new ideas or solutions I might have missed and clearing away old thoughts that are no longer relevant.

Talking to myself helps me get my thoughts in order, but I've also learned to appreciate the value of silence. I like to find a quiet place that I can simply experience the original state of nature in peace. Sometimes this ends up in me falling asleep, but more often it's a much-needed escape from the rigmarole of everyday, worldly affairs. When I find a quiet place both within myself and in my surrounding environment, I like to meditate, although I meditate when I am in locomotion also. Meditating helps me connect with the Supreme Energy. Even doing it for just a few minutes rejuvenates me. This is a big change from how I felt before the

---

[1]   "Healthy Aging." Johns Hopkins Medicine. https://www.hopkinsmedicine.org/health/healthy_aging/healthy_mind/the-power-of-positive-thinking

cancer treatments. When I would try to mediate when I was younger, I got bored quickly—it felt like it was a waste of time, sitting in silence and doing nothing. I've come to appreciate the benefits of meditation, though. I sit in silence and imagine a bright light covering my entire body, filling me with Its energy. After five minutes, a sense of peace and calm washes over me. When I finish, I feel as though I've just awakened to a cool, soothing sunrise.

This was experienced when I started going deeper into the Raja Yoga meditation practice, encouraged by the Brahma Kumaris World Spiritual Organization. My first time at one of their centers was when I attended a 'Diwali' celebration in October 2016. I got a profound understanding of the unique elements of us souls –we are energies filled with innate divine powers and virtues, having a great potential to amplify the truth within ourselves. Taking into consideration the similar attributes in various religious and spiritual entities, to the Divine Energy, the Source, or "God", I realized there is this unlimited ocean of light with which we can connect to operate from a basis of love for the self and all the situations around us. This bond with the Light has inspired me to stay consistent with my practice of self-improvement and of increasing values of cooperation, honesty, and benevolence. With this awareness, I check and shift my intellect in the direction that I feel is positive and purposeful as I understand the law of karma – what I sow is what is reap. Now, all that matters is that we amplify and live from our inner light.

Positive achievements can do a lot to increase your happiness, as well. When I'm sad or lonely I try to improve my skills in something I enjoy doing. I like to dance a lot, so often I'll work on devising a new step, or learning steps from other artists. Sometimes I'll record a video and share it with my friends. I play chess with my dad every day, and when I'm gearing up for a competition I'll focus on studying different chess moves, aiming to add another victory to my file. While I prefer winning, I'm often even more motivated by failure. Failure pushes me to keep growing and improving, never getting complacent with what I've already achieved. If I feel less self-confident, I read about the successes and failures of great figures from the past, and this gives me motivation to continue with my life.

I'm not the kind of person who ever feels bored anymore. I don't think it's ever true that there's nothing to do. You can always find something to occupy your time. If nothing else, you can explore your own creativity. I have a lot of hobbies, but sometimes when I have free time I prefer to draw and paint. I'll draw things that I like, or make up my own designs. There's an idiom that says, "An empty mind is the devil's playground," and there's some truth to this assertion. If your mind is occupied on a purpose, it doesn't have time to wander to dark places.

Just like positive thinking, creativity has medically proven benefits for both the physical and the mental health. In a 2015 article in *Psychology Today*, Dr. Cathy Malchiodi stated that it was her opinion creativity "may be as important to your health as balanced nutrition, regular exercise, or meditation."[2] She compiled over a hundred different studies on the link between health and creativity. Across the board, the results were conclusive. Engagement with the arts makes it easier to have a positive outlook—it decreases depression, reduces stress, and boosts your feeling of accomplishment. It can even boost your immune function. Dr. Malchiodi's study isn't the first to look into the link between being creative and improving your health. This is something that people have felt was true for a long time that is finally being verified by medical science. If you're taking an inclusive mind/body approach to your health, an emphasis on creative thought is one important aspect.

Some people simply aren't creative types and don't have any desire to paint, sculpt, make music, or take other similar outlets. Anything that engages your intellect will serve the same purpose, though. I like taking a topic I don't know much about and figuring out how it works. It doesn't matter whether it's a simple pen or something as complex as a system in the human body. The simple act of processing new information keeps your mind active. When you're feeling down or bored, finding even a small thing to distract you can bring you back into a more positive space.

During my chemotherapy, my dad would often sit beside my hospital bed and research the nutritional value of different foods. He'd study what combinations of ingredients would help me to stay healthy and saved recipes that looked especially appealing. He'd also find different ways of keeping me hydrated before and after my treatments. By focusing on these details instead of what I was going through, he didn't dwell in the negative thoughts of worrying about me. It ended up being a very practical use of his time, too. He made many of those recipes for us back home, and used the information about hydration and nutrition together to make me healthy juices, with things like celery, cucumber, and spinach. This was a lot better nutritionally than buying the pre-made, bottled green juices, which are often loaded up with sugar and lose a lot of the vitamins and minerals that would be in the raw fruit. I have to admit they weren't necessarily the tastiest concoctions; he'd add lemon or ginger to improve the taste, but each sip was still often hard to swallow. I made myself drink them, having heard him praise their health benefits.

I enjoy learning things about lots of topics. I especially like learning about nature, like animals and botany, and about history and food. I enjoyed visiting Hershey Chocolate Factory even when I was feeling tired or

---

2   Malchiodi, Cathy. "Creativity as a Wellness Practice." Psychology Today, 31 December 2015. https://www.psychologytoday. com/us/blog/arts-and-health/201512/creativity-wellness-practice

sick from the chemotherapy treatments, mostly because it was a chance to learn more about chocolate and how it's made. Even if the factory was done giving tours for the day, we would go to the Hershey Hotel and enjoy the surrounding area.

Surviving cancer has taught me never to lose hope. I think it's important that everyone set a goal and tread toward it, step by step. Setting a goal makes the positive outcome more tangible. When you can see where you want to get to as an end point, it's easier to lay down stepping stones to reach it. I truly believe that setting a goal also pulls that energy from the universe, calling its invisible power to your aid in its subtle, helpful ways.

I used to play basketball with my brother in between my chemo sessions. Even though my body didn't have much strength, I would still try taking jump shots. I never wanted to let my cancer keep me from going on. The same was true of my dance. I didn't want the weakness of my body to keep me away from the things I wanted to do, so I had supervised dance practices with Sujata Didi, Dr. Ram Goel's daughter, to keep my passions alive. Because I refused to let the illness dictate my life, I was able to keep in good enough form to prepare for a performance shortly after the end of my chemotherapy. If you never give up, success will find a way to reach you.

Another huge lesson I learned going through cancer treatments was to try and find joy in everything I do. I've always found school work to be a source of pleasure. I get a great sense of accomplishment when I'm able to tick an important task off of my daily to-do list. I get the same pleasure out of dance practices. Even when I'm tired or don't feel especially like dancing, I can get some satisfaction out of knowing that it's making me stronger and more fit. I try to enjoy the process and the journey for what they are instead of only thinking about the end result, but getting good results is enjoyable, too—an extra benefit when you've already gotten so much out of the learning process. Seeing its value also means that your efforts are never wasted. Even if the outcome seems to be a failure, you've at least learned a lot along the way.

When you fail, you simply discover one way not to accomplish your goal. It guides you closer to achieving it by process of elimination. As Thomas Edison famously said, "I have not failed. I've just found 10,000 ways that won't work." It's the eventual success you'll be remembered for, not any failures you faced on your way to getting there.

To approach failure in this productive way, I think you first have to be confident in your own strengths and abilities. I am very proud of myself—not only for surviving cancer, but also for all the other many accomplishments I've earned in my young life. I know I can achieve whatever I put my mind to. This abundant confidence has opened a lot of channels for me to try different activities without being afraid that I'll fail at them. Trying new things might let you find something that's even better-suited to your talents than the activities you're accustomed to. I joined classes in a variety of fields when I was younger: French language, painting, dancing, chess, golf, lawn tennis, and swimming, just to name a few. I didn't know I would be good at chess until I learned how to play it. Eventually, I reached the national level of competition for chess, became the captain of my school's team, and helped to represent them at the State Nationals in 2015. I never would have had that experience if I wasn't so eager to try new things.

I try to keep the same open mindset about criticism that I have about failure. If you use criticism to improve, it ends up being more valuable than a complement. I definitely learned this during my classes and studies of kathak. I had an inborn passion for dance and decided to develop this at Pracheen Kala Kendra Chandigarh, a renowned institution of art and culture in Northern India. My teacher there helped me develop my choreography by pointing out the things I wasn't doing as well so I would know where I needed to improve— something that can be hard to tell about yourself, especially with a physical art form like dance.

After I'd spent some time developing my dances, I decided to start recording videos of myself and uploading them to YouTube. I started with a cover of "Sun-Saathiya" from the movie *ABCD*. Now that I look back at it, it wasn't a very good performance—in fact, I think it might have been my most ridiculous performance on that song. I can't really blame myself since it was my first video. I checked back often for likes, views, subscribers, and comments. The "likes" and "dislikes" were about even and there were some negative comments, but I didn't let that bother me. I continued on with the next video in the series, "Manwa Laage". I choreographed the song myself, using a few steps I'd learned from watching Bharat Natyam, incorporated in with the kathak steps I'd recently learned in my classes. It ended up being one of the best recordings I made during that time span.

If I was frustrated by criticism or negative comments, I might not have continued with my dancing when things got difficult, and may have stopped posting videos after my first attempt. Instead, I used the criticisms to grow, and now have a YouTube channel full of videos, with over 25,000 views. My friends get impatient when I don't post a video for too long and always want me to upload more of them. I consider myself a budding YouTube artist, and while I'm still learning how to use the video camera and editor to give me a higher production value, I hope that my videos can inspire upcoming dancers. As an added benefit, dancing is excellent physical exercise. It helps me maintain my good health on many different levels.

YouTube has been a fantastic resource for developing my passion in dancing. I find it very motivating to watch other dancers like Elif Khan, Kinga Malec, Sonali Bhadauria, Pooja & Aparna and "Team Naach", just to name a few. There are even videos of classical personalities like Pali Chandra and Geetanjali that I can watch and learn from. I can experience and study whatever new dance forms I'm interested in, without waiting for my teacher to instruct me in them. YouTube acted as a vent for my frustrations when I was not taught the level of dance and the styles of dance I was capable of learning, thus expanding my creativity and versatility. I have the chance to play around with new things and take my time uploading new videos, letting myself enjoy the process.

Putting myself out there by uploading my dance videos to YouTube gave me the power to accept myself for who I am. I can depict my own style of dance, with as many videos as I want to make. I get a huge sense of pride out of doing my own choreography. It's a lot of work and responsibility, and I've learned by doing it that I'm capable of much more than I ever realized.

While I've always been interested in kathak, my passion for it has grown over the years. I have been a disciple of Dr. Samira Koser for about a decade now—more than half my life. Dr. Koser is herself a disciple of the acclaimed dancer Dr. Shobha Koser, from the Jaipur house of Kathak. I started studying with Dr. Koser at Pracheen Kala Kendra when I began taking lessons there, and much of what I learned about the dance form I owe to her. A few years ago, I attended a weekend workshop run by Ms. Aditi Bhagwat, a trained lavani and kathak dancer based out of Mumbai. I had learned of the workshop from my dear neighbor, Mrs. Neeta Sood, after I attended a dance program put on by Ms. Aditi Bhagwat and her troop in Tagore Theater. She had incredible agility. I learned a few of the basic Lavani steps and later practiced to learn them by heart.

Tagore Theater is one of my favorite places to watch performances—plays and music as well as dance. I especially remember one show put on by a Bengali artist Shobit Sen that was a one-man performance of music and drama. My father didn't want to go with me at first—he thought it would be boring—but when I insisted he tagged along. It ended up being a very memorable event. Tagore Theater is also where Pracheen Kala Kendra had put on its annual show, depicting the evolution of Kathak. In the group dance along with others, I presented Lucknow House of Kathak. The most exciting thing about this performance for me wasn't the dancing, but instead when I got the chance to see how the recording of music was being made. There was a staff member in the room with me who was overseeing the mix and recording. Dr. Koser was performing with a tabla artist as accompaniment. I sat down there in my general frock suit with my notebook, watching them, while Dr. Koser took the mic in her hand. Sometimes she told the tabla artist to play certain kinds of beats while she sang, the whole room filling with wonder thanks to her voice and the music. It was an amazing opportunity to get some insight into the studio recording process. I had to leave early to go to my tuitions, but I will never forget the things I experienced in the studio that day.

In early 2017 I was able to attend another workshop, this one led by the acclaimed Kathak expert Guru Malti Shyam, a disciple of Kathak maestro Pt Birju Maharaj, who dances in the Lucknow house. This house in particular interested me because it had a different kind of grace to its movements and body spins, how the whole stage is covered, so I was especially eager to attend this workshop. It was a three-day workshop, though I would have to leave for Delhi on the last day because I would be catching a flight from there to the United States, but I was sure I would still get to experience most of the workshop—a very exciting proposition.

The first day of the workshop, Guruji greeted me with a warm smile. She had a calming aura that instantly set me at ease. I will never forget the first lesson she taught me; whenever I take the first stance of a dance I should stand like I'm 2-3 inches taller than I really am. This was especially great advice for me, since I'm on the short side, but it's about the lines of the body and the projection of confidence more than it is for the sake of height. Since she taught me this trick, I started doing it even during practice. She was constantly telling me to smile throughout the workshop—another thing that was important for projecting confidence. By the end of the second day I was sad that I would have to leave early. Guruji commented that I had improved in my performance on the second day compared to the first, and know I could have learned even more if I was able to stay the entire time. I definitely left with my chin held high, far more confident in my skills than I'd been when I started. Even better, guruji invited me to stop at Kathak Kala Kendra to attend a few classes the next time I was in Delhi. It felt wonderful to know I'd created a bond with guruji in the two days of the workshop.

I think about achievements and happy memories like these whenever I'm stressed out. Having a zeal for life can help speed up the healing process—this is something that's been shown to be true by scientific studies, but you don't need a study to feel that it's true in your heart. Loving your life with all of your heart is one of the best ways to stay healthy. It's also true that happiness is multiplied—and sorrow divided—by sharing with others. I feel it's my duty to release good vibes into the world around me, helping to share my cheer and joy with anyone who may need it.

I try not to think about life in terms of positives and negatives, but instead to simply accept things as a part of life, because not everything that is negative in the moment will be negative in the long-term. Obviously I'm much happier now that the cancer treatments are over, not so much because of the discomfort of the treatments, but in terms of my health and the positive outlook I now have. The treatment removed all the worn-out cells from my body, letting new, fresh ones to be born. Once I'd recovered, I felt like a new baby who's just realized what the body is supposed to feel like even my eyesight improved. Before chemotherapy I'd worn glasses. After, I asked a family friend who was an eye specialist in Pennsylvania, Dr. Richard Lanning, if I still needed to wear my glasses.

"If you really feel you need them, you can," he told me. "But I don't think it's necessary."

Everyone was a bit bewildered to see me without my glasses. They kept asking me what the cure had been. I just told them it was magic, enjoying the looks that would get me.

The fact that I'm more conscious of my body's needs is a large part of why I'm healthier now than I was before the cancer treatments. This is a change anyone can make; you don't have to wait until something like cancer forces you to change your habits. My dad maintains a rigorous daily routine of nutrition and health, steering me away from junk food toward fresh fruits, vegetables, and juices, and making sure I get to bed at a reasonable time every night. Even when he's not around, I understand the importance of good health much better than most people my age. I don't let myself succumb to the temptation of violating this routine. I've started to actually enjoy this lifestyle. It feels like a natural part of my being. That's what happens when you form such a strong habit; it stays with you, and eventually doesn't even feel like it takes any effort.

The world is a wonderful, colorful thing, full of opportunities. If I am positive and excited about the possibilities of my future, these opportunities will come my way; by continuing to monitor my health, I'll be physically ready to seize them when they come around. Whatever challenges I face in the years to come, I know that I have the strength to overcome them. I will continue to live my life, my way, making the most of the years I have ahead of me.

Whatever challenges I face in the years to come, I know that I have the strength to overcome them. Even though I may not suffer physically from "Cancer", it can still present itself in other extreme forms of mental instability. My aim is to constantly maintain inner peace and to be constantly pulled by a fortunate future. I will continue to live my life, my way, making the most of the years I have ahead of me.

Printed in the United States
By Bookmasters